"For anybody on the road to serious weight reduction, these are important things to know."

> Paul Barrett Obis
> *Vegetarian Times*

"Paul A. Stitt has an exciting message for people who are tired of counting calories."

> Linda Fedak
> *The Columbus Dispatch*

Dear Friends,

I have started using your "Miracle Menu Plan," and in two weeks I lost 10 pounds. Have not found them again as with other plans, (smile). I am very pleased with how I look and how I feel, (smile). I have tried many other plans unsuccessfully, yours is really working miracles for me."

Thanks for introducing me to a plan that really works.

> Ledora K.
> St. Louis, MO

Dear Mr. Stitt,

I have just finished reading your book and I am so impressed by it that I would like you to send my parents the book for their anniversary. I feel that this may be the best present I can give them (better than any silver or gold!)

> Ann Marie V.
> Chicago, IL

Dear Mr. Stitt,

I recently read your new book, "Why Calories Don't Count," and was much impressed by it. Actually you advocate virtually the same method I used several years ago to lose 30 pounds without even trying.

> Loyd F.
> Leavenworth, KS

Dear Paul,

Since reading your book, I have changed my diet, eliminating 'white' flour and sugar as much as possible. I used to buy 5-6 candy bars and eat them all at once. I am thin but craved sugar. It took me a long time to convince myself it was bad for me. And I have exercised for a long time now — averaging an hour's walk 6 to 7 days a week. Thank you for your help.

Pat M.
Green Bay, WI

Dear Paul,

I know that personally your book and products have had a tremendous impact on my life and I am eternally grateful to you. I have changed my eating habits completely, and I feel great! I feel like I'm alive again.

Maurice B.
Milwaukee, WI

WHY
CALORIES
Don't
COUNT

BY PAUL A. STITT
WITH SCOTT KNICKELBINE

A Natural Press Paperback Original

WHY CALORIES DON'T COUNT

A Natural Press Paperback

Copyright© 1982
Second Edition 1983

by Paul Stitt with
Scott Knickelbine

Natural Press
A Division of Natural Enterprises
P.O. Box 2107
Manitowoc, WI 54220

Printed in the United States of America

Distributed by Contemporary Books, Inc., Chicago

Library of Congress
Catalog Card Number 82-80457

ISBN 0-939956-05-5

DEDICATION
To all those who want to feel
better and weigh less.

To Lorraine ;
Best of Health
to you.
Paul A Stitt

TABLE OF CONTENTS

FOREWORD

by Dr. Robert Mendelsohn
Author,
CONFESSIONS OF A MEDICAL HERETIC and MALEPRACTICE: HOW DOCTORS MANIPULATE WOMEN

Diet books are almost always about numbers; modern doctors are in love with numbers. They delight in counting. They are entranced by statistics. They regard quantification as synonymous with proof. They revere the objective numbers—which they call "hard" data—over subjective, qualitative values, which they derogate as "soft."

This fascination with numbers would not bother me if it improved patient care. Yet, over the last one-half century or longer, exactly the opposite has occurred. Whenever doctors have turned to numbers, people have been damaged. My own specialty—Pediatrics—provides many examples.

Babies have been damaged even before they are born, by the irrational belief of obstetricians in a magical number of pounds a pregnant woman "is allowed" to gain. Obstetricians have pulled different numbers at different times right out of thin air (10, 15, 25 pounds), seducing pregnant women into starving both themselves and their babies, mouthing inanities like "We want you coming through this pregnancy looking like a model." Models may be beautiful—but premature, low birth-weight babies are not. For at least two decades, scientific journals have carried impressive data relating maternal weight restriction to infant prematurity. Indeed, the recipe for creating prematurity—with its high infant mortality and its resultant intellectual deficit and neurologic damage—consists of quantitative maternal weight restriction. Modern doctors have yet to learn that the *quality* of the pregnant woman's diet is the crucially important—indeed, the only important—factor.

After the baby is born, the pediatrician, using fallacious growth tables, decrees that a baby has gained too many or too few pounds. Using the calibrated infant formula bottle, he prescribes exactly how many ounces a baby may or may not drink. He doesn't care about the quality of that bottle's contents—the high lead content, the absence of enzymes vital to the proper development of the human brain, the low vitamin B6 and mineral levels of some formulas, the cancer-producing potential of the nitrosamines present in the rubber nipples. Mesmerized by the numbers game, he is unconcerned about the millions of mothers and babies he has robbed or the historically and scientifically proven benefits of breast feeding. The infant scale and calibrated nursing bottles are his toys—objective, real, factual, proven, "hard."

An anxious mother phones the doctor about their sick child. Does the doctor first ask questions designed to elicit the nature of the symptoms, the common-sense description of the illness? Hardly ever. Why should he resort to the subjective, the qualitative, the "soft," when he can instead move into his fantasy world of numbers as he blurts out the catechism he has learned in his medical school seminary— "What's the temperature?"

Yet how many cases of severe meningitis have been missed because the doctor was lulled into a false sense of security by the fact that children with this potentially fatal disease often have "normal" temperatures? Conversely, how many tons of unnecessary, dangerous medications have been prescribed because the physician, panicked by a high fever, failed to consider the *quality* of the child's behavior and the all-important subjective symptoms, which could have lead him to the correct diagnosis of common, innocuous infant roseola?

Recently, the public has been given a peek into the bizarre world of doctors' counting, so that many people now know the major inaccuracies of the medically-worshipped standard height/weight tables. People are learning about the doctors' manipulation of the definition of high blood pressure, which automatically converts million of healthy citizens into patients dependent on doctors' treatments. Parents have recently caught the first glimpse of the hidden immunization statistics, including the true body count from whooping cough vaccine, one of the best-kept secrets of modern medicine.

The public is learning, painfully but speedily, that whenever doctors begin to count, patients had better run for their lives.

Paul Stitt's book now reveals that doctors—and their fellow-travelers in the field of establishment nutrition—threaten the lives and health of patients in yet another quantitative way: the counting of calories. Doctors have been trying for decades without success to evaluate nutrition by assigning numbers to calories—and fats, proteins, carbohydrates, vitamins, trace minerals, etc., etc. While the numbers keep changing, the goal—proper nutrition—remains for doctors as elusive today as it was a half a century ago.

Stitt effectively destroys the mythology of establishment nutrition. Yet the iconoclasm of *Why Calories Don't Count* is accompanied by invaluable, common-sense, authoritatively documented, easy-to-read, convincing advice—with emphasis on *quality* and kind of food. The sections on "Nutritional Density" particularly should be required reading for every medical student in every U.S. medical school.

But, realistically, we know that medical students are too busy being brainwashed into the numbers game to learn anything about nutrition other than to memorize the automatic response, "Just eat a well-balanced diet." Of course, if you want to find out what doctors mean by a "well-balanced diet," just look at hospital food! Or gaze at the pediatricians' illicit romance with Jello!

Since doctors are unlikely to read this book, patients must. Calories don't count, but Paul Stitt's landmark publication does. In a field marked by large quantities of error, this book glows with the quality of truth. For those of you who have abandoned one diet after another and discarded one book after another, take heart. Follow Paul Stitt's advice and this will be the last book on nutrition you will ever have to read!

Robert S. Mendelsohn, M.D. June 1982

INTRODUCTION:
Forget Diets!

Do you really want to lose weight?

Then forget calories! Forget carbohydrates! Throw away all those calorie charts and food scales and diet books! Ignore all the so-called "quick reducing" plans pushed by the latest crop of diet doctors! There's a better, healthier, more reliable way to drop those excess pounds and keep them off forever!

What's more, I want you to forget those terrible experiences you've come to associate with dieting. I want you to forget about the constant weakness you feel, the irritability and lack of concentration. And most of all, I want you to forget about *hunger*—the constant, gnawing hunger you feel after eating skimpy, unsatisfying meals; the hunger that ensures you'll eventually quit your diet and start to gain weight again.

I know what you must be thinking. All these years you've been told to keep careful track of the calories or the carbohydrates you eat. You've tried to carefully measure every mouthful, and check it against complex charts. You've become preoccupied with mathematics, desperately trying to keep your calorie or carbohydrate total below that prescribed by Atkins, Stillman, Tarnower, or the USDA. Now I'm telling you to ignore all those things, and you're confused. Doesn't dieting *have* to be complex?

You've also come to think of dieting as a very disagreeable experience. You think it's normal to feel famished on a diet—who wouldn't? After all, you get nothing to eat but a little lean meat, maybe a few spoonsful of mushy vegetables (if your diet allows any vegetables), perhaps a slice of flavorless white bread (if bread isn't a no-no). That's certainly not enough food to keep an adult happy. And you're *not* happy. You're hungry and tired and irritable, but you think that's how things have to be if you're going to lose weight. So it puzzles you when I tell you that you can feel full and happy and fantastically energetic, and still reduce. Doesn't a dieter *have* to be miserable?

The answer to both questions is a joyous, thundering NO! You don't have to be a math professor (or even a biochemist) to lose weight. And you don't have to feel hungry and irritable in order to have a slim, sexy, vibrant body. You just need to learn some simple truths about food. You must find out what your body really hungers for, and how to satisfy it—with a minimum of calories. Once you learn these things, you'll understand how everybody can lose the weight they need to lose, without feeling hungry and without fooling around with calories or carbohydrates.

The truth of the matter is that most calorie-or

carbohydrate-based diets reflect gross misunderstandings about how the human body works and what it needs. Many of the most popular diets are bad for you; others are foolish, and a few are downright dangerous. Almost all leave you hungry, and most create serious nutrient deficiencies which rob the body of energy and can lead to disease and even psychosis.

But the biggest problem with the average weight reduction diet is that, for most people, *it simply doesn't work*. Either dieters lose their will power and go off the plan long before they've reached their goal, or they stay on the diet until they're at their desired weight and then go back to their bad old eating habits and begin gaining again. As a result, most people are heavier one year after they begin a diet than they were when they started!

As worthless as most diets are, it's easy to see why people keep on trying them. Obesity in some form today afflicts over half of all Americans. And obesity does more than make us unattractive—it's killing us. The death rate for overweight individuals is substantially higher than the rate for individuals of normal weight![1] The evidence of obesity-related sickness is all around us. Our death rate from heart disease is more than double what it was at the turn of the century, and deaths from cancer have increased nearly three times in the same period.[2] No wonder more than 30 million Americans are now on a diet![3]

Two facts, then, are indisputable: First, Americans desperately need to lose weight. Second, calorie- and carbohydrate-based diets aren't helping them reduce. Where can the dieter turn for help?

I've written *Why Calories Don't Count* to teach you the few basic facts you need to know to start shedding pounds today. At the same time, you'll feel healthier and more filled with energy than you've ever felt before...and actually save money on your food bill! I've drawn upon my years as a food scientist to show you the underlying fallacies behind most diets, and to give you my own simple, natural method for easy weight reduction.

In *Why Calories Don't Count*, I'll reveal:

*The insidious inaccuracies in most calorie and carbohydrate charts—mistakes that keep you from losing weight.

*Why no one can tell you how many calories you really need.

*Why no amount of calories alone will ever satisfy you. . .and what your body is really looking for from food.

*The truth about *nutritional density*, a little known principle that will help you reduce and still feel great.

*The forgotten nutrient that fills you faster and actually reduces the calories you absorb from food.

*How hidden food addictions can sabotage your diet—and a simple way to free yourself from them!

I'll show you a special rotation diet to aid you in breaking your food addictions, and I'll even give you my popular *Miracle Menu Plan*, an easy seven-day meal schedule that has helped hundreds to lose weight and get back on the road to better health.

I promise you this book will change your mind about dieting. If you're on a diet right now, I'll show you the way to overcome those hunger pangs and that tiredness you're feeling. If you're not on a diet, but need to reduce, I'll give you a way to trim down that's not only effective—it's fun, and good for you! No matter who you are, no matter how much you want to lose, read on. . . and start today to build a slimmer, healthier, happier you!

NOTES

[1] Arnold E. Bender, *Nutrition and Dietetic Foods* (New: Chemical Publishing Co. Inc., 1973) p 84.

[2] "Average of Annual Death Rates for Selected Causes," 1980 *Information Please Almanac* (New York: Simon and Schuster, 1979), p 810.

[3] Bender, p 84.

1

THOSE MISLEADING CALORIE CHARTS:
They Can Trick You Into Extra Pounds!

An alarming number of myths and fallacies lurk behind today's diets. Some of the things many people think they "know" about dieting are disastrously wrong. Many of these misconceptions underlie even the basic methods that are commonly used in weight reduction plans. I want to start exploding some of those myths right now. Let's begin with a look at the most bothersome aspect of any diet: those pesky calorie charts!

You know the old routine. You fill your supper plate, estimate the size of serving of each food, and then check your handy chart to determine how many calories you're getting. It might run like this:

Your meal tonight consists of 1 lean pork chop, 1 cup of mashed potatoes with milk added, 1 medium tomato in slices, l cup of skim milk, and a fig bar for dessert. Sounds like an average meal. How many calories are in it? The answer— or *answers*—will shock you!

Let's select at random two different sources of calorie information. First, we'll check the United

States Department of Agriculture's Home and Garden Bulletin No. 72, *Nutritive Value Of Foods*. Then we'll look at the calorie listing in a typical diet book, for instance *Dr. Brennan's Diet Menus*.

We'll examine our sample menu from the bottom up. According to the USDA, 1 fig bar contains 50 calories.[1] But wait a minute. . .Dr. Brennan's book says that fig bar contains 60 calories.[2] That's a 10-calorie difference. . .but perhaps it's not too important.

We find more discrepancies in the rest of the menu. The USDA lists the cup of skim milk at 90 calories,[3] while Dr. Brennan lists it at 85.[4] And the tomato contains 40 calories according to the USDA,[5] while Dr. Brennan says it has 55—a 15 calorie gap.[6] It's when we come to the big items in our meal, though, that the differences become very disturbing. The USDA lists the cup of mashed potatoes at 125 calories,[7] but Dr. Brennan lists it at 165.[8] And the pork chop—USDA says it has 130 calories,[9] but Dr. Brennan says 285![10]

When we total up the calories, the results are truly stunning. According to the USDA listings, our sample meal contains 435 calories. But according to Dr. Brennan's listings, the meal contains 650 calories—a difference of more than 200 calories in one meal! A person using the USDA listing could even have another pork chop and still be under the calorie total of a person using Dr. Brennan's figures. How could the two calorie counts differ so wildly? Which one is right?

In fact, *both are probably wrong*. Now, I'm not accusing the USDA or Dr. Brennan of dishonesty or incompetence. We would certainly have found the similar discrepancies if we had compared other calorie charts. What's more, I'm sure they're all prepared with precise measurement and stringent scientific protocol. But even the most exacting methods cannot hope to overcome a single, unavoidable truth: *It is impossible for any calorie chart to give you an accurate idea of the number of calories in the food you eat!*

There are several reasons for the inherent inaccuracy of calorie charts, and some of them have to do with the qualities of the foods themselves. The plants and animals from which we draw our food are all biochemical individuals, and no two are alike. The amount of vegetable sugar in our tomato, for instance, will depend on its breed, the quality of the soil in which it grew, its growing season, and the amount of rainfall it got. Similarly, the amount of protein and fat in a pig's body is determined by its genetic inheritance, what it's fed, how much exercise it gets, and what hormones and other chemicals it has been exposed to. So you see, no two tomatoes ever contain the same number of calories, even though they may weigh the same. Nor will two pork chops ever be equally fattening. In fact, the caloric value of individual servings of the same food can differ quite drastically.

Aside from the inaccuracies caused by biochemical differences in foodstuffs, calorie charts can also be thrown off by differences in the precise quantities of food tested. Precisely how much meat is on an average pork chop? How large is a medium tomato? There's no way for scientists to determine these things with any accuracy, so they simply guess. And there can be no guarantee that the tomato you pick up in the produce aisle weighs the same as the tomato the USDA scientist tested.

The calorie chart listings for processed foods are even more misleading. Each food manufacturer determines how much sugar, fat, and starch it adds to its products, guaranteeing that virtually none of them are alike. For instance, the USDA says that a cup of peaches in heavy syrup contains 200 calories.[11] But Del Monte lists its peaches at 170 calories a cup, and Food Club lists them at 190 calories a cup. According to the USDA, green peas contain 115 calories a cup,[12] while Green Giant sweet peas list at 110 and Food Club at 120. The government says a slice of soft white bread contains 140 calories,[13] but Wonder Bread says two of its slices have 150. Clearly laboratory-produced calorie charts can give you no accurate information about the calories you're getting from processed foods.

It's easy to see, then, that the creation of a calorie chart is pretty much a hit-or-miss undertaking. But let's not blame the scientists for all the problems calorie charts create. You're partly responsible yourself!

Not that anyone could blame you. No one has the time or the equipment to make accurate measurements of the food he eats. When you have a juicy steak or a fresh apple in front of you, you want to eat it, not weigh it! And when you go out to eat, the last thing you want to do is start picking your dish apart and slapping it on a diet scale. So, you just give your food a look and try to estimate as best you can. Your estimates are probably seldom accurate, however, and your mistakes often add up to hundreds of uncounted calories.

And let's admit it. It's easy to cheat on all those measurements. When you're suffering from the hunger and weakness most dieters live with, it's easy to turn your teaspoons of sugar into heaping teaspoons and your cups of milk into "generous" cups. If the measurements are all inaccurate anyway, why not err on the side of satisfaction?

When you consider all the things that can go wrong in calorie measurement—biochemical differences in food, difficulties in scientific measurement, fluctuations in the caloric content of processed foods and errors (intentional and unintentional) that dieters make themselves—it's not difficult to see why counting calories accurately is a nearly impossible job. Even in a controlled experiment, with scientific measuring devices and strict controls, keeping track of calories is a sloppy affair.

You might ask, "What's wrong with a little inaccuracy?" More than you might think! The problem is that the inaccuracies build up, and can lead to excess pounds. An error of 5 percent (about the difference between the USDA and Green Giant's estimates for a cup of peas) maintained over an entire year could lead to a 15-pound weight gain, and the errors in our sample meal above could lead to 156 excess pounds a year! Luckily for us, our own bodies keep us from making such astronomical errors. Nevertheless, these calculations serve to show that reliance on calorie charts can actually work against you in your efforts to lose weight.

I'll bet those of you on low-carbohydrate diets are feeling pretty smug and congratulating yourselves for avoiding the calorie trap. But really, you're in no better shape than the calorie counters. In fact, carbohydrates are even more difficult to count than calories! A calorie is simply a measure of heat given off when a food is oxidized by the body—or just burned in a calorimeter. But a carbohydrate is a complex chemical composed of carbon, hydrogen and oxygen. Carbohydrates are the sugars, starches, gums and cellulose, and these can only be measured through chemical analysis. Further, carbohydrate charts are prone to most of the same inaccuracies as calorie charts.

A quick glance at two popular carbohydrate guides will prove my point. The *Complete ABC Carbohydrate Diet Guide* says that a banana has 23 grams of carbohydrate,[15] while *Carlton Fredericks' Calorie & Carbohydrate Guide* puts the figure at 26 grams—about a 12 percent increase.[16] The ABC guide lists a two-inch slice of angel food cake at 22 grams of carbohydrate,[17] while Fredericks' guide lists a six centimeter slice (a little over two inches) at 32 grams.[18] Carbohydrates are no easier to keep track of than calories, and weight loss on a low-carbohydrate diet can be just as difficult.

The point I'm trying to make is this: foods are not mathematical values that nature produces in standardized units; they're real things. Good food is alive, growing and dynamic. Processed junk food is subject to modification at the whim of the processers. Either way, food cannot be neatly quantified. Although your body can accurately detect the nutrient content of the food you eat, a food scientist can only do an inaccurate, unreliable job.

So who are you going to trust? Your own body, or some guy in a white coat?

NOTES

[1] United States Department of Agriculture Home and Garden Bulletin No. 72, *Nutritive Value of Foods* (Washington: U.S. Govt. Printing Office, 1971), p 28.

[2] Richard O. Brennan, *Dr. Brennan's Diet and Menus* (Irvine, California: Harvest House Publishers, 1978), p 156.

[3] USDA, p 5.

[4] Brennan, p 122.

[5] USDA, p 18.

[6] Brennan, p 126.

[7] USDA, p 17.

[8] Brennan, p 166.

[9] USDA, p 11.

[10] Brennan, p 162.

[11] USDA, p 22.

[12] USDA, p 16.

[13] USDA, p 25.

[14] Roger J. Williams, *Biochemical Individuality* (Austin, Texas: University of Texas Press, 1956), p 159.

[15] *Complete ABC Carbohydrate Diet Guide* (North Miami, Florida: Merit Publications, Inc., 1972).

[16] Carlton Fredericks, *Carlton Fredericks' Calorie and Carbohydrate Guide* (New York: Pocket Books, 1977), p 173.

[17] *ABC Guide*, p 6.

[18] Fredericks, p 181.

2

MISSION IMPOSSIBLE
Determining Your "Caloric Need"

As hopeless as it is, counting calories is just the first half of a luckless ritual that all dieters must perform. For at the same time they're totaling calories, they're also making sure the total stays below some magic figure that they've been told is their caloric need for the day. They've read in the diet books that people have to eat a certain number of calories a day to maintain their body weights. All you have to do to find *your* caloric need is to look it up in a chart in the back of your diet book. Then (so the story goes), all you have to do is eat less than the number of calories shown in the table and the weight will start melting off, right?

Wrong again! In reality, those charts that tell you how many calories you need are every bit as misleading as the charts that are supposed to tell you how many calories you're getting. In fact, for many people, eating even an amount substantially less than their recommended daily calorie intake will make them *gain* weight! How can that possibly happen?

In order to see how eating less than your

"caloric need" can make you heavier, let's examine the first question every dieter asks: What's my daily caloric need? The answer: it depends on whom you ask, and when you ask them!

The most widely accepted source for caloric allowances is the National Research Council of the National Academy of Sciences, so we'll focus on the NRC's figures. Suppose you're a 23-year-old female who weighs 55 kilograms (120 pounds). How many calories do you need each day to maintain your body weight? If you had asked this question in 1966, the NRC chart would have told you you need 2025 calories a day.[1] However, since 1974, the NRC has suggested that 23-year-old, 120-pound females eat only 2000 calories a day.[2] The differences for a male are even more glaring. A 23-year-old man who weighed 70 kilograms (154 pounds) was told in 1966 that he needed 2900 calories a day to maintain his body weight.[3] Today, however, he'd be told he needs only 2700—200 hundred calories fewer each day![4] These calorie differences are important. If we convert them into possible pounds gained (basically, by dividing by 3,500) we see that if our woman, who only needs 2000 calories a day (by current estimates) was actually eating 2025 calories a day (as 1966 NRC figures told her to), she could gain as much as three pounds a year. Her twin brother would be in bigger trouble, though. If we assume today's NRC figures are correct (and there's really no reason to, but we'll get to that in a minute) we find that by eating the 2900 calories per day allowed in 1966, he'd gain up to 21 pounds a year! And remember, the NRC is constantly revising these figures DOWN. What will your "caloric need" be next month? Next year?

You needn't dabble with mathematics to see how inaccurate such "caloric need" charts can be. Just talk to the people you meet every day. One close friend of mine says that if she eats the NRC-prescribed 2000 calories a day, she gains weight very quickly. A man I know was surprised to find when he went on a diet containing 20 percent fewer calories than his "caloric need" that he was eating more food than before he started the diet! And we all know folks who gain weight on a low-calorie diet. In fact, statisticians have noted that obese people on the average eat LESS than slim people![5]

One of the most fascinating studies I've ever read was done by marketing researchers at Philip Morris, Inc. They were collecting information on middle-aged male smokers and non-smokers. The survey happened to include questions on body weight and eating behavior. In analyzing the information, the Philip Morris researchers made a startling discovery: caloric intake did not increase with increasing levels of obesity. In fact, the researchers concluded, "The results of the study agree with other studies cited in failing to find a direct relationship between overeating and obesity."[6]

Why are estimates of caloric need such poor

indicators of how much you should eat to maintain or lose weight? The answer lies in an all-important concept: *biochemical individuality*. Each of us, indeed every organism on the face of the Earth, is a biochemical individual. The shape, size and capacity of every organ in your body, and the rate and precise nature of every chemical reaction going on in your cells, is unique to you. Your body and its functions are shaped by your special genetic inheritance. It is biochemical individuality that knocks all the caloric need charts into a cocked hat, because it reveals that there is no "average" caloric need or any "normal" rate at which food energy is converted to fat.

An important factor which determines how much weight you lose or gain is your *basal metabolism*. Basal metabolism is the minimum energy you must expend for the maintenance of respiration, circulation, digestion, body temperature and glandular activities. It is the least amount of energy you must have in order to live. For any further activity, of course, your energy needs increase. Basal metabolism is influenced by age, health and body weight, as well as genetic inheritance. Now, the problem with charts purporting to show your caloric need is that they are all calculated in terms of a single, average basal metabolism rate, usually 1 calorie per kilogram per hour for men and 0.9 calories per kilogram per hour for women.[7] How likely is it that your basal metabolism is average?

Not likely at all! In fact, your metabolism

could be significantly higher or lower than the "average." In a restricted-diet experiment conducted by the Carnegie Institution, metabolic information was gathered on groups of healthy male adults. The study showed that, even for men with identical body weights, basal metabolism—and thus caloric need—varied by as much as 50 percent![8] As a matter of fact, basal metabolism for normal individuals may vary by even wider margins, with very few falling within the average range.

This biochemical individuality in basal metabolism has serious consequences for the calorie-counting dieter. For instance, suppose you're a 24-year-old woman who weighs 128 pounds. The NRC says you need 2000 calories to maintain your weight, so you decide to go on a weight-loss diet of 1500 calories. You are assuming that by eating 25 percent less than your caloric need, you'll start to lose weight. But now assume that your basal metabolism is 50 percent lower than the average, so your real need is only 1000 calories. If your metabolic rate is unusually low, you may be obese, even though you may eat no more than your slim friends. You'll actually gain weight on this "low calorie" diet!

What's more, individual features of your metabolism may differ from an imagined "norm." For instance, your body may tend to process carbohydrates into fat at a faster rate than most individuals. If that's the case, your caloric need may be substantially lower than the figures you read in charts. The truth is that metabolism is a complex process, and it is never precisely the same in any two people. No chart can ever tell you your real caloric need.

Another factor that throws caloric need charts off is exercise rate. Obviously, a person who is very active and who expends a lot of energy will need more calories than an inactive person. But most caloric need charts are based on only one level of activity, called "moderate." It's clear that such a chart is as useless to the accountant as it is the the lumberjack; neither could be considered "moderately active." Some charts try to get around this by including several activity levels, but these are usually vague and arbitrary. For example, one chart constructed by Marvin Small in *The Easy 24 Hour Diet* has caloric need listings for Inactive (does nothing actively), Mildly Active (rides to work, sits at work), Medium Active (teacher, mother of small children), Active (on the move most of the time) and Very Active (physical worker plus extra exercise)[9] It's difficult to see where many individuals would fit in such a scheme.

Consider a friend of mine, a writer. He rides to work, and spends most of his day sitting in front of a word processor. However, he runs a mile every day, is a Frisbee enthusiast, and stays fairly active on weekends. What category does he fit in? Surely his exercise program makes him too active for the Mildly Active category. But is he active enough for the Medium Active slot? He's not a teacher, and he's certainly not the mother of small children! This chart won't be much help to him. The description of Active individuals is confusing as well. What does it really mean to be "On the move most of the time?" Does it describe an assembly-line worker or an executive who spends her day rushing from meeting to meeting? And what about the Very Active category? How many physical laborers do you know who get (or even need) more exercise on the side? With all these questions unanswered it seems pretty clear that even this five-category chart is unable to give us a clear idea of how our activity level translates into calories. Each of us has his or her own special activity level, which changes from day to day and from year to year. Trying to squeeze yourself into a category can only lead to mistakes—mistakes that can work against you as you try to lose weight.

Individuality is really the key to the failures inherent in the low-calorie or low-carbohydrate diets. Biologically we are individuals, and we each have our own special life-styles. When you consider that we are each different in our genetic backgrounds, our health, our metabolisms, and the level of exercise we get, you begin to understand that a chart drawn up by some scientist in a laboratory setting really has little to do with the number of calories you burn every day. This is an important point: the charts listing caloric need, like the charts claiming to give the caloric content of foods, are more than simply inaccurate. They are *irrelevant*.

In the end, there's only one person in the entire world who can determine how much you must eat to maintain or lose weight. And that's you.

NOTES

[1] Bogert, Briggs and Calloway, *Nutrition and Physical Fitness* (Philadelphia: W.B. Saunders Company, 1966), p 79.

[2] Corinne H. Robinson, *Basic Nutrition and Diet Therapy* (New York: Macmillan Publishing Co., Inc., 1980), p 72.

[3] Bogert et. al., op. cit.

[4] Robinson, op. cit.

[5] Theodore Berland and the editors of *Consumers Guide, Rating the Diets* (New York: Rand McNally & Company, 1974), p 196.

[6] Berland, p 17.

[7] Bogert et. al, op. cit.

[8] Roger J. Williams, *Biochemical Individuality* (Austin, TX: University of Texas Press, 1956), p 120.

[9] Berland, p 181.

3

DIET DISASTER:
You've Got A One-Way Ticket!

So far we've been talking about the technical problems concerning low-calorie or low-carbohydrate diets. Calories are impossible to count accurately. No chart can show you your caloric need. In light of these two problems alone, losing weight by counting calories is an extremely difficult task. Studies have indicated that only one-tenth to one-quarter of people on calorie-restriction diets succeed in losing more than 25 pounds, and almost all dieters are back to their original weights within a year or two! Calorie counting simply doesn't work for most people!

You may be thinking, though, that the problem is simply a technical one. Suppose we could find a way to determine the precise caloric content of every food that we eat. Suppose too that every individual could determine exactly how many calories he or she should eat to lose weight. With all the technical problems out of the way, shouldn't the low-calorie or low-carbohydrate diet work?

Theoretically, yes; realistically, no. It is a fact

that overweight is caused by consuming too many calories. If an organism really restricts its caloric intake, all other things being equal, it will lose weight. But it is also true that an individual who wants to lose weight and stay slim must consistently maintain lower calorie consumption... *forever*. And it is this final truth that delivers a knockout punch to most low-calorie diets.

In the first place, while some people are willing to tolerate the annoyance of calorie-counting for a few weeks, very few will put up with it for the months it takes to lose significant amounts of weight, and almost nobody wants to count calories for the rest of his or her life! But more importantly, most low-calorie diets are extremely unpleasant. Comic writer Art Buchwald has gone so far as to declare that the word "diet" is a form of the Latin verb "to die!" It is quite common for people on diets which emphasize calorie-watching to experience weakness, irritability, constipation and constant, grinding hunger. It's very hard for most of us to live with hunger for even a day; who wants to live with it forever? As a result, most dieters cheat on their diets or give them up completely, and soon gain back all the weight they may have lost.

The majority of people simply can't stay on a low-calorie diet for the rest of their lives. Why not? The answer lies in the mechanisms which control the body's need and desire for food. To understand why calories don't count, we must look within the body itself.

What causes hunger? Many dieters are convinced that it's a lack of calories that makes them hungry. It's not hard to understand why they think so; it seems to them that when they eat all the calories they want, they feel full, while when they go on a low-calorie diet they feel hungry. But the truth is that *your body does not count calories*. You can eat many more calories than you need and still feel hungry. On the other hand, it is possible to eat far fewer calories than you eat now and feel full and satisfied.

An eye-opening experiment done in New York in 1977 revealed some fascinating evidence that the body does not count calories. A group of obese patients checked into a hospital and were given a practically unlimited supply of food. Their time at the hospital was divided into six periods. During the first two periods, the food they were given contained a normal number of calories. During the second two periods, however, the sucrose in their food was secretly removed and replaced with aspartame, a non-nutritive sweetener. Thus, without the subjects' knowledge, the caloric value of their food was decreased. During the final two periods the subjects received normal food once again. The subjects' food intake and body weights were carefully monitored.

Now, if the body were satisfied by calories, we would expect the subjects' food intake to increase as its caloric value decreased. Surprisingly, though, the experiment showed very different results. Even though the caloric content of the food decreased during the second two periods, the subjects' food consumption remained constant. Even though the subjects ate as much as they liked, they actually lost weight! When the caloric value of the food was returned to normal, consumption still remained stable? The subjects' bodies were not counting calories. Instead, they were looking for something else in their food.

Well, if the body isn't looking for calories, what IS it looking for? Science is still not sure. Scientists feel that hunger is largely controlled by an area   of the brain they call the appestat, which is believed to be located in the hypothalamus, at the base of the brain. But little satisfactory scientific study has been done to determine what triggers the appestat. Some feel it's looking for blood sugar, others think it's looking for fatty acids. Yet there is little firm evidence to support these theories. Not only are specific body functions difficult to isolate, but the methodology for studying hunger often consists of surgically tampering with the gastrointestinal system, injecting nutrients into the stomach or damaging portions of the hypothalamus of test animals. Such drastic measures make it hard to tell if observed behavior truly reflects normal body function. Besides, the sensation of hunger itself is almost impossible to measure objectively. Reliable answers are hard to come by.

Yet we do have some clues as to what triggers and satisfies hunger, although these clues are often overlooked by biochemists.

One important clue is witnessed today most often in the animal kingdom: *Animals tend to balance their own diets*. Fascinating studies have been done in which animals were provided with unlimited amounts of a vast variety of raw nutrients. When the animals are healthy, they invariably eat the proper amounts of all vitamins, minerals, and other nutrients (without once consulting a Recommended Daily Allowance chart). Adult human beings today less frequently show this ability to self-select their diets, both because of the extreme nutrient imbalances in their bodies as well as the brainwashing they get from television every night. But studies done with young unspoiled children show that they too will naturally select a nutrient-balanced diet[3] It seems clear that organisms tend to hunger for a balanced nutrient load.

The second important clue is one we experience every day: *cravings*. I first came in contact with this phenomenon as a boy. My younger brother was constantly putting gravel in his mouth! Try as they might, my parents couldn't get him to stop. Finally we learned that he had a serious calcium deficiency; without being conscious of it, my brother was seeking to correct the deficiency with the most calcium-rich "food" at hand!

Doctors have long noted that significant nutrient deficiencies make us hungry for certain kinds of foods. One of the most common cravings is for peanut butter. Doctors find that those who crave peanut butter also happen to be deficient in the B vitamins; not surprisingly, peanut butter is a rich source of the B complex. People who take diuretics or cortisone often crave bananas, which are rich in the potassium these drugs rob from the body. And habitual apple-eaters frequently are short on calcium, magnesium, phosphorus and potassium. Anyone who's had these or other cravings knows first-hand that nutrient deficiencies can make you hungry.

It is important to distinguish between those occasional cravings which signal the body's need for some nutrient, and the constant craving of a *food addiction*, however. One is a natural, healthy bodily signal and the other is the result of the body's metabolism distorted by some toxin. I'll explain more about food addictions in Chapter 6.

The ability of animals—and humans in the natural state—to self-select a balanced diet, and the phenomenon of cravings: both are vivid examples of the body reaching out, not for calories, but for vitamins, minerals and other micronutrients. I believe that only one conclusion is possible in light of such evidence: *The body is hungry for all nutrients, not just for carbohydrates, proteins, and fats.* Conversely, if your body is significantly deficient in some micronutrient, you will be hungry, *no matter how many calories you've consumed!* Thus the important factor your body looks for from foods is not calories, but quantities of macro- and micronutrients. I call this factor *nutritional density.*

There are two other factors which help to "turn off" your sensations of hunger. The first is the amount of chewing you must do to eat a food, and the second is the physical content of your stomach. Scientists feel that the mouth plays an important role in satiety: the more you have to chew, the more satisfied you are; your brain recognizes that your mouth has done enough work for one meal. Also, while you're chewing, your body has time to recognize the presence of nutrients which will cause the appestat to signal fullness.

More important still is the physical content of the stomach. Your stomach can sense how much food it contains. When it contains enough, it sends fullness signals to the brain. Biologists are not quite sure just how this happens. Some feel that the stomach has nerves (called mechanoreceptors) which sense the tension of the stomach walls. More recently some have theorized that the stomach contains receptors (called chemoreceptors) that react to the presence of nutrients in the stomach. The fuller the stomach is, the more of these chemoreceptors are exposed to the stomach contents, and so the more fullness signals the brain receives. Either way, the physical bulk of the stomach contents does influence satiety.

Luckily, there is one nutrient which quickly satisfies both the need of the mouth to chew and the need of the stomach for fullness—*fiber*. Fiber is the portion of fruits or vegetables which is not broken down in the stomach. Fiber is usually contained in the skins and seeds of these products, and makes them both chewy and bulky. Fiber from many sources (bran, for instance), also tends to absorb digestive juices in the stomach and thus produces even greater volume. Thus dietary fiber is a crucial factor in making you feel full.

So we now have two parts of our fullness equation: nutritional density and fiber. These are what the body looks for from food. These are what it hungers for; these are what will satisfy it. A diet high in these two factors will produce satisfaction, health, and weight loss. A diet low in them will produce only hunger, sickness and possible weight gain. Next to nutritional density and fiber content, caloric content is a very small matter indeed.

Now that we understand the hunger equation, it's easy to see why the average low-calorie diet produces such terrible side-effects and ultimately fails for most people. Let's look at three typical meals included in a medically-approved reducing diet:[4]

Breakfast ½ cup orange juice
1 boiled egg
1 slice toast (usually from white bread)
Tea or coffee

Lunch   1 frankfurter
            1 roll (usually from white flour)
            Celery and radishes
            Tea or coffee

Dinner   3 ounces of roast beef
            1 cup spinach (probably boiled)
            ½ cup carrots (again, boiled)
            Tea or coffee

Now, what can we notice about this typical diet? Immediately we can see that these meals contain far less food than most people usually eat. Now that we understand what causes hunger and what satisfies it, we know that, for this diet to work, it should contain plenty of nutrients and fiber to create a feeling of fullness and well-being. But does it?

Not at all! In the first place, many of the foods in this sample diet are very low in nutritional density. The white flour products, for instance, are robbed of most of their essential vitamins and minerals ("enriching" puts back only a few, and some of these cannot be used by the body), yet contain high levels of calories and carbohydrates. The vegetables, too, if prepared the way most Americans prepare them, will have significant amounts of their nutrients boiled out of them. The only foods on the menu high in nutritional density are the raw vegetables at lunch, but these will probably be eaten in too small a quantity to make much difference. It would be hard to get enough vitamins and minerals from a diet like this if you could eat all you want; the skimpy portions in this weight-reducing diet, however, provide dangerously low amounts of nutrients.

How about fiber, the other factor in our satisfaction equation? This sample menu contains *almost no fiber whatsoever!* Breakfast is fiber-free, save for the tiny amount in the white bread, which has had most of its fiber removed. The celery and radishes are providing almost all the fiber at lunch, and boiling in water reduces the fiber-per-serving of the vegetables (mostly because you're getting more water per cup). And of course the meat in this diet contains no fiber at all.

Low nutrients and low fiber; that combination in this diet almost guarantees it will fail. But that's not all! There are ingredients in this diet that actually *stimulate* hunger! The boiled egg, the frankfurter, and the vegetables will probably be served up with salt...a proven appetite stimulant. That hot dog also contains nitrites, MSG, and other chemical additives designed to whet your appetite. The white flour products almost certainly contain fat and sugar, both sure to make you ravenous for more.

And the caffeine in all that tea and coffee! Many diet plans recommend tea or coffee for two reasons, both misguided. First, neither contains any calories by itself. Second, as a stimulant, caffeine is a temporary appetite depressant. But what the diet books never tell you is that caffeine interferes with sugar metabolism and contributes to chronically low blood sugar—hypoglycemia—which in turn leads to weakness, irritability, and hunger. Yet this doesn't stop low-calorie diet advocates from telling you to drink all the coffee, tea and sugar-free cola you want.

Actually, this sample diet is not an exceptional case. ALL diets that consist of processed food not only will fail to fill you, but will actually *increase* your hunger. This is because America's food conglomerates are out to sell you hunger, not satisfaction.

It's easy to see why the production of foods that make you hungry is good for the food industry. After all, the less satisfying a product is, the more of it you'll tend to eat. The more you eat, the more you must buy. The more you buy, the more you pay out to the food companies. So the food companies get bigger, and you get fatter (and sicker). This is why processed foods are invariably of low nutritional density. They also have as much fiber as possible removed, because the food industry realizes that, as Dr. David Reuben has pointed out, "The low-roughage diet literally compels overconsumption, making obesity almost *inevitable*."[5] (I explain more about the food industry's conspiracy to sell you hunger in my book *Fighting The Food Giants*.[6] It doesn't bother the food industry that the low-nutrient, low-fiber garbage they turn out leads to obesity, heart disease, diabetes, hypoglycemia, colon cancer, schizophrenia, etc. etc. What matters to them is that you eat more food.

Now, it's bad enough to suffer the many

diseases that result from a regular diet of processed, nutrient-robbed, addictive foods. But for the dieter, it's even worse. He must live on minimal amounts of this junk forever if he's going to lose weight and keep it off the low-calorie way. The result: *diet disaster.*

The first and most pervasive outcome of a low-calorie processed food diet is severe nutrient depletion and metabolic distortion. Even the United States government admits that it is simply impossible for an individual on a 1000 to 1200 calorie-a-day diet to receive even the barest minimum nutrient requirements.[7] When the body does not get the nutrients it needs, it must draw them from its own limited stores. Once these run out, and in most cases even *before* they run out, the individual suffers organ damage, and begins to show deficiency diseases.

Such rapid nutrient depletion leads to a severely distorted metabolism. Denied the scores of substances needed for hundreds of delicate biochemical reactions, the body can no longer successfully turn foodstuffs into energy or organ tissue. In fact, such metabolic distortion can in many instances make it almost impossible to lose weight or keep it off, despite the meager caloric content of the diet that brought on the distortion.[8]

Nutrient depletion strikes most cruelly at the brain, your most sensitive organ. And it is just such depletion of the brain's nutrient stores which is responsible for one of the prime symptoms most dieters show: extreme irritability.

The B-complex vitamins, so important for good nervous system function, are not adequately provided by the processed food diet. As the brain runs low on these and other important nutrients, the individual grows nervous, indecisive and easily upset.

A University of Minnesota study demonstrated the devastating effect of the low-calorie processed food diet on mental health. Thirty-six healthy men, none of them overweight, were put on a 1500 calorie-a-day diet for six months. Although none of them suffered any overt physical illness, all of them sustained significant psychological deterioration. They became tired, irritable, apathetic, antisocial, and lost interest in women. Some suffered such severe deterioration that they were taken off the diet; the rest exhibited neurotic symptoms for an extended time after the test.[9]

As serious as these mental symptoms are, the low-calorie processed food diet leads to many physical ailments as well. All the body's organs suffer from the drastically warped metabolism low most diets bring on. As a result, junk food dieters are prone to heart disease, arthritis, kidney failure, gall-bladder disorders and cancer. The low fiber content of the processed food diet also contributes to the constipation many dieters experience, as well as diverticulosis and diverticulitis, colitis and colon cancer. Dieting on processed foods is not only a bad idea; it's positively dangerous!

As frightening as the health effects of a

processed food diet are, the most damning
symptom of such a diet is more simple, and more
pervasive: *hunger*. Robbed of nutrients, eating
little or no fiber, individuals on the low-calorie
processed food diets are constantly hungry.
They walk everywhere with a gnawing in their
stomach. They become obsessed with food. They
dream about it. Eventually, the torment becomes
unbearable. They cheat on their diet, then they
give it up altogether. They gain back the weight
they lost, and weeks later they are even heavier
than when they started. Their diet has failed.

* * *

Have I frightened you? Good. You need to know that most low-calorie diets are nonsense—lethal nonsense.

But I would not have presented such a horrifying picture of today's calorie-obsessed diets if I weren't absolutely sure there's a better way. And there is! You can begin to lose weight easily and effectively, and still feel great.. in fact, feel more vibrant, sexy and alive than you've ever felt before. I know of a diet plan that you'll love, a diet that will have you wondering how you could ever eat the way you're eating now.

Want to learn more about this amazing yet simple method for effective weight loss? Read on!

NOTES

[1] Arnold E. Bender, *Nutrition and Dietetic Foods*, 2nd. Ed. (New York: Chemical Publishing Co. Inc., 1973), p 86.

[2] Katherine P. Porikos, Glenn Booth and Theodore B. Van Itallie, "Effect of covert nutritive dilution on the spontaneous food intake of obese individuals: a pilot study," *The American Journal of Clinical Nutrition*, 30: October 1977, pp 1638-1644.

[3] Roger J. Williams, *Biochemical Individuality* (Austin, TX: University of Texas Press, 1977), p 159.

[4] David Reuben, *The Save Your Life Diet* (New York: Ballantine Books, 1975), p 98.

[5] Ibid.

[6] Paul A. Stitt, with Mark Knickelbine and Scott Knickelbine, *Fighting The Food Giants* (Manitowoc, WI: Natural Press, 1980).

[7] Theodore Berland and the editors of Consumers Guide, *Rating The Diets* (New York: Rand McNally & Company, 1974), p 180.

[8] E. Cheraskin and W.M. Ringsdorf, Jr., with Arline Brecher, *Psychodietetics* (New York: Bantam Books, 1974), p 29.

[9] Cheraskin and Ringsdorf, pp 29-30.

4

NUTRITIONAL DENSITY:
The Secret to Effective Weight Loss

Now that I've thoroughly disillusioned you about calorie-counting diets, it's time we start learning a new way to eat, a way to stay constantly full, healthy and satisfied, and still lose weight. It shouldn't surprise you that, just as our satisfaction equation (remember, *nutritional density + fiber = satisfaction*) showed us why most diets fail, the same equation can show us how to construct the perfect diet. Let's start by examining the first factor in our equation, *nutritional denisty*.

What exactly is nutritional density? Simply put, nutritional density expresses the quantities of important nutrients a food contains as compared to the amount of food energy (calories) it delivers. So a food that's low in calories and high in nutrients is said to have a high nutritional density, while a food that's high in calories and contains only moderate or small amounts of nutrients is said to have a low nutritional density. Since the dieter wants to feel satisfied and healthy while cutting down on calories, it follows that he or she must eat nutritionally dense foods.

Luckily, you don't have to be a biochemist to discover foods which are the most nutritionally dense. You don't even have to consult a chart, although I do provide nutritional density listings at the end of this chapter. All you need to know is that there is one type of food that always delivers the greatest nutritional density: *natural foods.*

What are natural foods? The term can cause a lot of confusion, because it's bandied about by so many people in the food business today, and not all of them use it honestly. When I say natural food, I mean food that has undergone the absolute minimum of processing. For most fruits and vegetables it means fresh and raw, or lightly steamed. Of course, some foods need a bit of processing before they're usable by the human body; potatoes and corn must be cooked to break down the starch granules, grain must be baked into bread, sprouted or ground into cereal. But in all instances, the amount of milling, cooking and manipulating must be kept to the absolute minimum. *No* natural food contains chemical additives or preservatives of any kind. *No* natural food contains added refined sugar or white flour, and *no* natural food is laced with any added flavor enhancers such as fat and salt. Most of all, natural foods must be whole foods; foods with every bit of the natural bran, germ, seed, skin or whatever left on. In short, natural foods are foods that are as close as possible to their natural state.

There are several reasons why natural foods

have high nutritional densities. In the first place, nutrients—especially the micronutrients—are very fragile things. Cooking heat, for instance, easily destroys thiamine, riboflavin, pyridoxine, vitamin C and many other vitamins normally found in fresh, raw food. Just the act of storing a food for a few days can reduce the potency of most of the B-complex vitamins, as well as folic acid. And according to vitamin and mineral expert Earl Mindell, the rough handling foods get as they're processed can destroy or hinder the absorption of practically every known micronutrient.[1]

Let's face it. . .our ancestors were wandering vegetarians for the most part, and the span of time between harvesting and consuming was usually very short. In the few tens of thousands of years since that time our food culture has changed drastically; fruits, vegetables and grains are stored for weeks or even months before they show up on the supermarket shelves, and by that time they have almost always been processed and overcooked. Even so, our bodies are still geared to that ancient hand-to-mouth existence, and we still need the vitamins, minerals, enzymes and other important growth factors found only in fresh, whole foods.

Secondly, as I pointed out in the last chapter, the whole thrust of the processed food industry is to make foods that won't satisfy you. One of the most effective ways to do this is to remove nutrients from food. Usually this is done by removing the parts of foods that contain most of the nutrients: the bran and germ from grains, the skin from potatoes and fruits, and the natural oils from vegetable products. The result of processing is food that you want to eat a lot of, *and this is precisely because it is of low nutritional density.*

It's easy to find examples of how processing robs foods of their nutritional density. Applesauce, for instance, contains only about half the phosphorus, potassium, vitamin A, riboflavin and niacin of fresh whole apples, and only 25 percent of the vitamin C. Yet applesauce has nearly twice the calories per 100 grams![2] Bread made with whole wheat has nearly four times the magnesium,[3] three times the phosphorus, more than twice the zinc, five times the vitamin B6 and substantially more folacin than "enriched" white bread. White bread does come out ahead in one category, though. . . calories.[4] Do a little nutritional detective work of your own, and you'll soon have all the proof you need that processed foods—even "enriched" foods—can't compete with whole natural foods for nutritional density.

When dieters look for nutritional density, then, they should look for natural foods. They pack the most macro- and micronutrients into the fewest calories. And that spells satisfaction...and easy, life-long weight control!

But some people find it difficult at first to switch to a natural foods diet. With all the media hype and the nutritional misinformation most of us have received since our school days, it's not always easy to make the wisest food decisions. So let me provide a few guidelines to help you on your way to natural weight loss:

BUY FRESH. Make sure the food you eat is as fresh as possible. Naturally, this means buying much of your food from the produce section of your supermarket, rather than from the canned food aisle. Try to find a store which makes every effort to get fresh produce, no matter what the cost. "Discount" fruits and vegetables have often been stored for months, and then treated with dyes and waxes to make them fresh-looking. Such "junk food" produce is often deficient in many vitamins, minerals and enzymes. The freshest food of all comes from your local farmers' market, or, of course, from your own garden!

When you can't buy fresh, buy frozen produce. Although freezing can destroy many micronutrients, it is less harmful than canning, which combines water and heat to remove much of the water-soluble nutrients in foods. You might even buy fresh food in season and dehydrate it yourself for longer shelf-life.[5]

EAT IT RAW. If a food can be eaten with no cooking, eat it that way whenever possible. As we've said before, cooking and boiling can destroy nutrients or dissolve them away. Thus a fresh raw unpared apple will deliver much more nutritional density than a baked apple or applesauce, and a big spinach salad will be more satisfying than a few spoonsful of mushy, boiled spinach. Besides, raw food simply tastes better!

If you must cook, be sure to lightly steam your fruits and vegetables, using as little water as possible. Microwaving vegetables with just a sparse covering of water is a good idea, too.

REDISCOVER BREAD. Good whole grain bread is a nutritionally complete food, and it should be at the center of any natural foods diet (unless you have formed a maladaptive reaction to it—see Chapter 6). Whole wheat bread not only provides a full range of micronutrients, but it is also a good source of protein and complex carbohydrates.

But be careful; many of the things you've been taught to look for in bread are in fact the things you should look *out* for. For instance, many people think that fresh bread should be soft and squishy. Wonder Bread ran a ludicrous ad campaign a few years back which sought to hoodwink consumers into believing that a bread should be judged by how much it can be squeezed. In fact, it is chemical additives which give the squishyness to Wonder and other processed breads, including some of the so-called whole wheat breads on the market, many of which contain very little whole wheat flour. A good bread is one that is firm, crumbly, and won't roll into a doughball in your hands. It should be chewy, and have a rich grainy flavor. All these signs indicate that a bread has as much of the whole grain as possible left in.

As you rediscover bread, cut down on meat, especially red meat. Meat is actually very high in fat and a very poor source of protein, and although it delivers a lot of the B-complex vitamins, whole grain products actually do a better job with fewer calories (and less cost, as well!)

READ THE LABEL. Give the packaged foods you buy a complete examination before you put them in your shopping basket. Pay careful attention to the lists of ingredients. If you see that the food contains any artificial additives, flavors, colors, stabilizers, emulsifiers, preservatives or spoilage retardants, pass it by. If it contains refined white sugar, corn syrup, dextrose, or high amounts of brown sugar, you can do without it. If it's made with refined flour (any sort of flour not specifically called whole-grain), leave it on the shelf. The best rule of thumb is: if you can't pronounce it, don't buy it.

It is especially crucial to avoid so-called "diet foods." Most people don't realize that manufacturers convert foods into diet foods primarily by reducing the over-all food value of the product. Thus some diet breads contain 50 percent fewer calories because they're sliced twice as thin. But at the same time, the bread contains 50 percent less of a whole range of nutrients. Similarly, other diet foods have their calories reduced through the addition of bulking agents, water or air—additives which can do nothing to satisfy you. Certainly, some of these are enriched, but we've already discussed how empty those claims of enrichment are.

To add insult to injury, many diet foods are made tastier with artificial flavor enhancers and salt, ingredients which will add fuel to the flame of your   all-consuming hunger. Diet foods are no dieter's friend!

One more extra-special word of warning: DO NOT, DO NOT, DO NOT DRINK DIET SOFT DRINKS. Almost all of them contain caffiene, which, as we said, is a potent appetite stimulant. I have heard grisly reports of unpublished weight-loss studies conducted at the University of Wisconsin. Some of the subjects drinking diet soda were said to have become so hungry they actually ate the flowers friends sent them! If you're thirsty, drink water. Amen.

START SLOW. Some people try too hard and too fast to convert to a natural foods diet. After years of a synthetic, chemically-laden junk food diet filled with bizarre textures and make-believe flavors, people need some time to adjust to the subtle taste and robust texture of whole, real food. Families with children especially need to take time to adopt a healthful diet. (Barbara Reed, who worked for 20 years in the criminal justice field has traced the profound effects leading children from a junk food diet to life as a criminal in her book, *Food, Teens And Behavior*.)

You might start by removing one junk item from your family's each day and replacing it with a natural food. Get rid of the coffee this week, and try one of the many wonderful varieties of herbal tea. Next week throw out the sugar and fat-loaded snack foods and replace them with sweet ripe fruit and mixtures of nuts, raisins and seeds. Gradually introduce whole grain breads at every meal, and start to cut back on meat. Try a new raw or lightly cooked vegetable each week. Experiment! Natural food can be more exciting than that processed garbage ever was!

Once you've replaced the processed items in your diet, you'll be well on your way to healthful, delicious eating and permanent weight control. The next step is to use body wisdom to modify your diet to meet your special nutritional needs.

What's body wisdom? It's the principle which acknowledges that your own body knows what it needs, and can tell you when it's missing something, or when it's getting something it can't handle. Remember the test animals in the last chapter who self-selected their own balanced diet? They were operating on body wisdom. Although humans naturally have as much body wisdom as any animal, we also have an ability animals don't have: the ability to be misled by advertising campaigns. We've been tempted to consume vast amounts of junk, and this silences body wisdom. Scientists have actually demonstrated that a prolonged processed food diet can warp an organism's ability to select a balanced diet for itself[6] This is why it's so important to return to a natural foods diet before we can begin to tell what nutrients we have special needs for.

And no doubt about it. . .each of us has his or her own nutritional needs. The concept of biochemical individuality, which we discussed in Chapter Two, applies every bit as much to vitamins, minerals and other micronutrients as it does to energy intake. A normal human's daily need for calcium, for instance, can vary from 3.52 to 16.16 milligrams per kilogram of body weight.[7] The B vitamin requirement for humans has been shown to vary over at least a four-fold range.[8] As a result, the Recommended Daily Allowance for nutrients as set by the National Research Council is really a poor guide to the amount of nutrients you need each day. There is only one authority on your body's nutritional needs, and that's you!

Once you've partially stabilized your metabolism by switching to a natural food diet, you must begin to be aware of the signals your body sends to let you know of some nutrient deficiency. Unusual physical symptoms—and some symptoms Western civilization has come to accept as normal—are often signs of deficiency. Here are some of the common ailments that nutrient deficiencies can cause. How many are bothering you?

Symptom	Deficiency
Appetite loss	Protein, Biotin, Phosphorus, Sodium, Zinc, Vitamins A, B1, or C.
Bad Breath	Niacin
Body Odor	Vitamin B12.
Bruising Easily	Vitamin C, Bioflavonoids.

High Cholesterol B complex, Inositol.

Constipation   B complex, Fiber.

Diarrhea   Vitamin K, Niacin,
                   Vitamin F.

Dizziness   Manganese, Riboflavin.

Ear Noises   Manganese, Potassium

Eye Problems   Vitamin A, Riboflavin.

Fatigue   Zinc, Protein, Vitamin A, B
                   complex, PABA, Iron,
                   Iodine, Vitamin C, D.

Gastrointestinal   Vitamin B1, B2, Folic Acid,
Problems   PABA, Vitamin C, Chlorine,
                   Pantohenic Acid.

Dandruff   Vitamin B12, F, B6,
                   Selenium

Loss of hair   Biotin, Inositol, Chlorine,
                   B complex.

Heart Palpitation Vitamin B12

High Blood   Choline
Pressure

Infections	Vitamin A, Pantothenic acid.
Insomnia	Potassium, B complex, Biotin, Calcium.
Loss of Smell	Vitamin A, Zinc.
Memory Loss	Vitamin B1.
Menstrual Problems	Vitamin B12.
Mouth Sores	Vitamin B2, B6.
Muscle Cramps	Vitamin B1, B6, Biotin, Chlorine, Sodium, Vitamin D.
Nervousness	Vitamin B6, B12, Niacin, PABA, Magnesium.
Nosebleeds	Vitamin C, K, Bioflavonoids.
Retarded Growth	Protein, Vitamin B2, Folic Acid, Zinc, Cobalt.
Skin Problems	Vitamin A, B complex.

If you suffer from any of these, your body is telling you of a serious nutrient deficiency. Sometimes cravings will tell you which foods to eat to meet such shortages. Today, however, with body wisdom so silent in most people, Mother Nature needs a little help from nutritional research. Here are some foods you might try to eat to meet vitamin and mineral deficiencies:

VITAMIN A
Fish liver oil, carrots, green and yellow vegetables, eggs, milk and dairy products, yellow fruits.

VITAMIN B1
Dried yeast, rice bran, whole wheat, oatmeal, peanuts, most vegetables, bran, milk.

VITAMIN B2
Milk, yeast, cheese, green leafy vegetables, fish, eggs.

VITAMIN B6
Brewers yeast, wheat bran, wheat germ, cantaloupe, cabbage, blackstrap molasses, milk, eggs.

VITAMIN B12
Eggs, milk, cheese.

VITAMIN B13
Root vegetables, whey.

VITAMIN B15
Brewers yeast, brown rice, whole grains, pumpkin seeds, sesame seeds.

BIOTIN
Nuts, fruits, brewers yeast, egg yolk, milk, unpolished rice.

VITAMIN C
Citrus fruits, berries, green and leafy vegetables, tomatoes, cauliflower, potatoes, sweet potatoes.

PANTOTHENIC ACID
Whole grains, wheat germ and bran, green vegetables, brewers yeast, nuts, blackstrap molasses.

CHOLINE
Egg yolks, green leafy vegetables, yeast, wheat germ, lecithin.

VITAMIN D
Fish liver oils, sardines, herring, salmon, tuna, milk and dairy products.

VITAMIN E
Wheat germ, soybeans, vegetable oils, broccoli, brussels sprouts, leafy green vegetables, spinach, whole wheat, whole- grain cereals, eggs.

VITAMIN F
  Vegetable oils, peanuts, sunflower seeds, walnuts, pecans, almonds, avocados.

FOLIC ACID
  Green leafy vegetables, carrots, tortula yeast, cantaloupe, apricots, pumpkin, egg yolk, avocados, beans, whole wheat flour.

INOSITOL
  Brewers yeast, cantaloupe, grapefruit, raisins, wheat germ, blackstrap molasses, peanuts, cabbage.

VITAMIN K
  Yogurt, alfalfa, egg yolk, safflower oil, soybean oil, fish liver oils, kelp, leafy green vegetables.

NIACIN
  Whole wheat products, brewers yeast, wheat germ, fish, eggs, peanuts, avocados, dates, figs, prunes.

BIOFLAVINOIDS
  Pulp of lemons, oranges and grapefruit, apricots, buckwheat, blackberries, cherries, rose hips.

PABA (Para-aminobenzoic Acid)
  Brewers yeast, whole grains, brown rice, wheat bran and germ, blackstrap molasses.

CALCIUM
Milk and milk products, all cheeses, soybeans, sardines, salmon, peanuts, walnuts, sunflower seeds, green vegetables.

CHLORINE
Salt, kelp, olives.

CHROMIUM
Shellfish, corn oil, clams, brewers yeast.

COBALT
Milk, oysters, clams.

COPPER
Peas, whole wheat, prunes, shrimp and most seafood.

IODINE
Kelp, vegetables grown in areas where the soil is iodine-rich, onions, all seafood.

IRON
Farina, raw clams, dried peaches, egg yolks, oysters, nuts, beans, asparagus, blackstrap molasses, oatmeal.

MAGNESIUM
Figs, lemons, grapefruit, corn, almonds, nuts, seeds, dark green vegetables, apples.

MANGANESE
Nuts, green leafy vegetables, peas, beets, egg yolks, whole grain products.

MOLYBDENUM
Dark green leafy vegetables, whole grains, legumes.

PHOSPHORUS
Whole grains, eggs, nuts, seeds.

POTASSIUM
Citrus fruits, watercress, green leafy vegetables, mint leaves, sunflower seeds, bananas, potatoes.

SELENIUM
Wheat germ, bran, tunafish, onions, tomatoes, broccoli.

SULFUR
Fish, eggs, cabbage.

VANADIUM
Fish.

ZINC
Wheat germ, brewers yeast, pumpkin seeds, eggs, nonfat dry milk, ground mustard.

Sometimes a person's special need for a certain nutrient will be too large to satisfy comfortably from food alone. This is a problem many people in modern society have, since our increased levels of stress and environmental pollution place nutritional demands on our bodies that our ancestors never experienced. Many individuals have especially large requirements of vitamin C and the B complex vitamins. In these instances, food supplements may be necessary. While I don't intend to get into food supplements in this book, I highly recommend that you do some digging for yourself. An excellent place to start is *Earl Mindell's Vitamin Bible* (Rawson, Wade Publishers, Inc.), a book from which I drew much of the information presented above.

As helpful as such advice from doctors, nutritionists and biochemists can be, *the key to using body wisdom is to listen to your own body*. Become aware of the sensations within you. Carefully note what the foods you eat do to you. Which foods truly satisfy you, and which make you hungry for more? Which make you feel alive and alert, and which leave you tired and irritable? Do certain foods make you "high?" Do you develop negative reactions or allergies to others? Only your own body can tell you these things. Listen to what it tells you, and act accordingly.

Once you've used body wisdom and natural foods to help you to a high-nutritional density diet, you'll be surprised at how easy and satisfying weight loss can be. You'll find that your food intake will taper off, but you'll never feel hungry. Your appetite for high-calorie processed foods will disappear, and you'll also get over any craving for alcohol you might have. Your metabolism will begin to normalize, and your weight will stabilize. If you're overweight, you'll start to slim down, and the weight will stay off.

And there are other benefits to be had from a nutritionally dense diet. You'll begin to feel better than you have in years! Those little aches and pains you thought you'd have for the rest of your life will disappear, and you'll have energy to burn. You'll feel so good you'll *want* to stay on the diet for the rest of your life...and a long life it will be, too!

To help you get started on your nutritional density diet, I've prepared a chart which lists foods on high nutritional density. Now, nutritional density is a difficult thing to measure and express. No calculation can ever be exact, and every method of determining nutritional density has some faults, mine included. But as a means of rough comparison, I believe my nutritional density table will give you helpful information as to which are the best high-nutrition/low- calorie foods.

NUTRITIONAL DENSITY

HIGH NUTRITION,
LOW CALORIE FOODS.

Eat as much of these as you want, provided you do not react to any of them.

Apricots
Asparagus
Beans, Green Snap
Beet Greens
Broccoli
Brussels Sprouts
Cabbage, Common
Cabbage, Chinese
Carrots
Cauliflower
Celery
Chard,
Swiss Collards
Cucumbers (unpared)
Currants
Dandelion Greens
Eggplant
Endive
Gooseberries
Grapefruit
Grapefruit juice
Guavas, Common
Kale
Kohlrabi
Leeks
Lemons

Lemon Juice
Lettuce, Romaine
Liver (Veal)
Mackerel, Atlantic
Mangos
Mushrooms
Muskmelon, Cantaloupe
Muskmelon, Honeydew
Mustard Greens
Okra
Onions
Oranges
Peas, Green
Peppers
Pumpkin
Radishes
Rutabagas
Spinach
Squash
Strawberries
Sweet Potatoes
Tomatoes
Turnips
Watercress
Wheat bran

SPECIAL PROTEIN FOODS.

Eat some at each meal.

Almonds
Avocados

Brazilnuts
Bread, Whole Wheat
Bread, Natural Ovens
Buckwheat, Whole Grain
Cashews
Cheese, firm natural
Chicken, White Meat
Cod
Corn
Crab
Dried Beans, all types
Eggs
White Fish
Filberts (hazelnuts)
Jerusalem Artichoke
Lentils
Lobster
Milk
Millet, whole grain
Oatmeal
Oysters
Peanuts
Peanut Butter (natural)
Peas (mature, split)
Pecans
Potatoes, with skins
Red Snapper
Rice, Brown
Rye, whole grain
Salmon
Soybeans
Soybean Curd (Tofu)
Soybean Flour

Sunflower Seeds
Turkey
Wheat, whole grain
Wheat Flour, whole
Wheat, Shredded
Wild Rice Venison
Yogurt

MODERATE NUTRITIONAL DENSITY.

Eat these occasionally.

Apricots
Apples
Bananas
Beef, lean
Blackberries
Boysenberries
Buttermilk
Cherries
Loganberries
Nectarines
Peaches
Persimmons
Pineapple
Raspberries
Waterchestnuts
Watermelon

LOW NUTRITIONAL DENSITY.

Eat only on special occasions, the less often the better.

Apples, peeled
Bacon
Cherries, sweetened
Corn, canned
Cranberries
Deep fried foods
Fruit Cocktail
Gelatin
Lamb
Molasses,
light Pears
Pineapple, canned
Pistachio Nuts
Plums
Pork
Potatoes, mashed
Potatoes, French fried
Prune Juice
Rhubarb (sweetened)
Shrimp, french fried

POOR NUTRITIONAL DENSITY.

Avoid whenever possible.

Beef, Chuck
Beef, Choice Sirloin
Beef, Hamburger

Bread, French & Vienna
Bread, Raisin
Bread, rye
Bread, White enriched
Candy
Canned vegetables
Commercial Cookies
Corn Flakes
Corn Grits
Cornmeal (degermed)
Crackers, Graham
Cranberry Sauce
Cream
Non-Dairy Creamer
Donuts
Jellies and Jams
Lamb
Lemonade (commercial)
Macaroni
Marmalade, Citrus
Milk, condensed
Olives, Green
Pickles
Pineapple (sweetened)
Potato Chips
Rice, White
Salad Dressing
Soft Drinks, powdered
Soda Pop
Sugar (brown and white)
Sweet Rolls
Tapioca
Tang

NOTES

[1] Earl Mindell, *Earl Mindell's Vitamin Bible* (New York: Rawson, Wade Publishers, Inc., 1979), pp 24-96.

[2] United States Department of Agriculture, *Composition of Foods* (Washington, D.C.: U.S. Govt. Printing Office, 1975), p 6.

[3] USDA, p 149.

[4] USDA figures reprinted in Tom Gorman, "Now we know—wheat does beat white...," *Bakery*, June, 1981, p 53.

[5] Mary Bell, *Dehydration Made Simple* (Salt Lake City, UT, 1981)

[6] Roger J. Williams, *Biochemical Individuality* (Austin, TX: University of Texas Press, 1956), p 161.

[7] Williams, p 137.

[8] Williams, p 152.

5

FIBER COUNTS

As important as it is in any effective weight loss program, nutritional density is only the first part of the satisfaction equation. There is another, equally important part: *fiber*. Your diet must provide both nutritional density and fiber if you are to feel full and satisfied, and lose weight at the same time. But before I show you how to increase the fiber in your diet, let's answer a few questions first. Why is fiber so important in human nutrition? What IS fiber, anyway?

As you recall from Chapter Three, fiber plays two crucial roles in satiety. First, it provides satisfaction by giving your jaw muscles plenty of work to do. The crunchiness and chewiness of high-fiber foods means you'll have to put out some effort in order to eat them. And, as we have seen, the amount of effort you put into eating helps determine how much you'll eat before you feel full. Foods which are easy to eat are also easy to over-eat.

Second, we said that fiber adds bulk to foods, and this bulk increases the volume of food in your stomach. As you remember, your stomach is very sensitive to the volume of its contents; as your stomach becomes fuller, it starts sending satiety signals to your brain.

In this chapter, though, we're going to go beyond our earlier discussion of fiber. We'll discuss how fiber works, and the many things it can do to help you lose weight and maintain general health.

Fiber comes from the cell walls of plants. Because the wall serves as a protector for the plant cell itself, it is very tough; extremely harsh acids which are not found in the human stomach. As a result, fiber itself is not digested or absorbed by thebody, but passes through the gastrointestinal tract more or less intact.

There are many types of substances which fall into the category of fiber. All are polysaccharides, meaning that they are complex structions of monosaccharides,or carbon-water molecules. Most important is cellulose, which is the prime constituent of the skeletons of most plant structions. It is extremely complex chemically, and breaks down only in the presence of strong acids. Then there is hemicellulose, which resembles cellulose in chemical structure but is more soluble and more easily broken down. Pectin is the name of a group of substances found in fruit. One of them is the familiar carbohydrate used in making jellies, but there are others as well. Various gums and lignin are also included in the fiber group. Each of these types of fiber behaves differently in the body, and each has its role in good nutrition. It is important that you eat a variety of high-fiber foods in order to get all of the types of fiber you need.

We have already seen that fiber helps restrict the amount of food you eat by filling your stomach faster. What else can fiber do for the dieter? Plenty. Most importantly, *fiber can actually restrict the amount of calories you absorb from food!*

You see, once fiber leaves the stomach, it mixes with the half-digested food in the intestines. This mixing accomplishes two things. First, since the fiber has not been brocken down into a mushy paste like the rest of the meal, it helps to keep the material loose and bulky rather than tight and compact. Second, since fiber tends to retain water, it keeps the half-digested material moist. As a result, a high-fiber meal moves more quickly through the small and large intestine than a low-fiber meal.

A meal's transit time through the gastrointestinal system is very important, because it is in the intestines that most nutrients are absorbed—including carbohydrates and other high-calorie materials. If the food moves slowly through the intestines, the body has time to absorb every last calorie from the food. If the food moves quickly through the intestines, however, calorie absorption is cut down, sometimes by 14 per cent or more!

This is why some Africans have been known to eat 3,000 calories a day—including six hundred grams of carbohydrates—without gaining a

pound[1] Their diet consists of unrefined corn,
beans, and other natural, high-fiber foods. As a
result, the food they eat moves swiftly through
their gastrointestinal systems (24 hours from
consumption to excretion, as compared to
three days for most Americans), and they never
suffer from obesity according to Dr. William
Dam of Fox Lake, Illinois who has worked in
Africa, the only fat Africans are those who have
switched to a low-fiber, American diet!

Perhaps now you can understand why fiber is
so important to anyone who wants to lose
weight. Medical findings about fiber completely
overthrow the notion that weight-watchers must
restrict themselves to skimpy meals. In fact, if
you're sure to get a high amount of fiber in your
food, you could actually eat *more* than you're
eating now and still lose weight!

But fiber can do even more for the dieter. It has
been shown that individuals on a high-fiber diet
tend to excrete more body fat through the bowel
movement than people on a low-fiber diet[2]
Thus a high-fiber diet not only prevents you from
becoming obese, but also actively works to
eliminate body fat.

A number of different types of fiber are
responsible for this fat excretion. Cellulose helps
absorb and bind dietary fat and carry it out of
the body. Lecithin and other materials in the
fiber family, such a pectin, act in the bloodstream
to dissolve fat and cholesterol deposits and carry
them away for excretion. A study in the early
'60s on black and white subjects in South Africa

showed that patients on a high-fiber diet excreted substantially more fat in their feces than did subjects on a low-fiber diet.[3]

You might say than fiber is a miracle nutrient for dieters. It makes foods more satisfying, so you eat less; it hustles food through the digestive trct so you absorb fewer calories; it helps the body excrete its own excess fat. Really, though, it shouldn't surprise you that dietary fiber can do so much to prevent obesity. After all, even before our earliest ancestors first started walking on two legs, they survived on high-fiber foods: fresh, whole fruits and vegetables. Over millions of years of evolution, the human body adapted to the fiber content of natural foods. Even today, our digestive systems still need the fiber content of a natural food diet to regulate food consumption and restrict calorie absorption.

My point is this: fiber does not "trick" your digestive system into being satisfied with less food or absorbing fewer calories. Rather, fiber helps your gastrointestinal tract operate *normally,* the way it was designed to. It is not normal for a human being to be fat. And with a high-fiber, natural food diet, you need never become fat or remain overweight.

Incidentally, a high-fiber diet can do a lot more for you than just help you lose weight. For instance, because it loosens waste material in the lower intestine, it effectively prevents constipation—a malady often suffered by calorie-counters on the traditional American processed low-fiber diet. If you eat plenty of fiber, your lower intestine is kept free of compacted waste matter, and this will prevent an entire array of "diseases of civilization" which currently plague westerners.

Colon cancer, for example, has been linked to the action of microorganisms naturally found in the gut upon the digestive juices, such as bile acid, in the lower intestine. If this fecal material is not eliminated quickly, the microorganisms excrete carcinogens into the bloodstream, and colon cancer—one of the most prevalent types of cancer in America today—is the result.

Hemorrhoids plague millions of Americans, and these too can be traced to our low fiber diet. Hemorrhoids are extremely distended veins in the anal region, caused by the great pressure an individual must exert to expel compacted fecal material from the colon. Contrary to the absurd popular belief, hemorrhoids are not caused by sitting! Instead, they are caused by the low-fiber processed diet most of us eat.

Compacted material in the lower intestine is responsible for other maladies, from diverticular disease to appendicitis, from colitis to varicose veins. There's no doubt about it—the intestinal sluggishness caused by our low-fiber diet is a dangerously unhealthy condition.

There's even another important thing this miracle nutrient, fiber, can do for you: *It can protect you from hidden poisons in the food you eat!*

This amazing preventative quality of fiber was demonstrated by an experiment at the

Institute for Nutritional Sciences in Los Angeles.

Scientists there were studying the toxicity of cyclamate sweetener.

The cyclamate was given to two groups of rats, each on a different diet. The first group ate standard rat food pellets, which are high in fiber. The second group ate a synthetic diet which was very low in fiber.

Within three days, the rats on the low-fiber diet began to show symptoms of cyclamate poisoning, and within two weeks all the rats in that group were dead. But the rats on the high-fiber diet were able to avoid nearly all symptoms of cyclamate poisoning.[4]

This same protective effect of dietary fiber has been demonstrated in studies of a number of other harmful drugs as well. Dietary fiber helps decrease the absorption of toxins from food, but the body has every opportunity to absorb toxins from low-fiber material which compacts in the lower intestine.

All the marvelous facts about the benefits of fiber could fill an entire book, and in fact many books have been written on the subject. If you want to learn more about how fiber works in the body and what it can do for you, I urge you to do more research on your own.

Now that you're excited about losing weight the high-fiber way, it's time you learn how to increase the fiber in your diet. And Rule One in any high-fiber diet won't surprise you at all: *eat natural foods.*

Why whole, natural foods? Because they

contain all those things that provide fiber—skins, hulls, seeds, bran, etc. These are precisely the parts of food that are removed by the food conglomerates, because they make food too filling. White bread is much easier to gulp down that whole wheat bread, and for good reason: whole wheat bread has four times the fiber of white bread. In fact, nearly all natural foods contain substantially more fiber than their processed counterparts. Whole apples have twice the fiber of applesauce, corn has more than twice the fiber of sugar frosted corn flakes, brown rice has three times the fiber of white rice. When you're looking for high fiber, just as when you're looking for nutritional density, look for natural foods.

A word of caution. Many people are becoming interested in dietary fiber, and the processed food industry is waking up to this interest. But leave it to the Food Giants to develop "high fiber" foods that still make you hungry! For instance, a certain bread manufacturer has introduced a bread with the ridiculous name "Whole White." They announce that Whole White bread is high in fiber, but is still soft and white and gummy, so people can eat a lot of it at a sitting. How do they do it? They take their fiber source—in this case pea bran—and grind it very fine. The resultant powder mixes completely with bread dough and doesn't change the texture at all.

Unfortunately, studies have shown that reducing plant fiber to a powder almost completely eradicates all of its beneficial properties.[5] Fiber must be long-grained, as it is found in whole fruits and vegetables and in stone ground whole-grain products, in order to function effectively in the digestive system. Any completely "invisible" fiber source is doing you no good at all.

How much fiber should a person get in a day? That's terribly hard to say. The average American gets perhaps 20 grams of dietary fiber a day, and suffers from obesity, colon cancer and heart disease. The average Zulu may get as much as eight times that amount, and suffers from none of these diseases. It would be easy to say "Well, then, try to get 160 grams of dietary fiber a day." Easy to say, that is, but hard to swallow. You'd have to eat the fiber equivalent of more than forty small apples a day to get 160 grams, and I don't thing very many Americans are ready for that. Besides, it's not clear that you need that much fiber to be healthy.

I believe that an American ought to get about 50 grams of dietary fiber a day to stay happy and healthy. It's quite easy and comfortable to maintain this level of fiber consumption. Many other nutrition-conscious doctors recommend similar daily amounts.[6] Of course you can always eat more fiber if you want to!

In fact, that's the beauty of counting fiber rather than counting calories or carbohydrates— *there's no danger in under-estimating.* You can eat 50 percent more fiber than you thing you're eating, and it will actually be good for you! When it comes to fiber, you can safely say "When in doubt, *eat more.*" Imagine saying that about calories!

How should you begin to increase the amount of fiber you eat? The first thing to do is eat natural, high-fiber foods. (I've included a listing of the fiber contents of dozens of foods at the end of this chapter.) Be sure that they are unprocessed. Eat plenty of raw vegetables and whole grain products. And if you really want to go high-fiber, cut down on the meat you eat. Fiber is a vegetable product, so meat has no fiber whatsoever. Remember: the more meat you eat, the less fiber you consume.

Be sure to get a good amount of fiber—perhaps 10 or 20 grams—at every meal. It will do you no good to try to cram down 40 grams of fiber at breakfast (for instance, by eating two cups of 100 percent Bran cereal) and then slacking off the rest of the day; your digestive system will slack off too.

It's also important to remember to start slowly as you increase your fiber consumption. Chances are your system has never dealt with more than small quantities of dietary fiber. It will need a chance to adjust to the greater volumes of high-fiber foods. Start by raising your fiber consumption to 30 grams a day. Next week, increase to 40 grams. Later, increase to 50 grams, 60 grams, and as far beyond as you feel comfortable. If you eat too much too fast, you'll feel uncomfortably bloated. Bowel movements could become painful, and you may even suffer a sort of backlash constipation. Easy does it! Even increasing fiber by small increments will do a great deal to help you lose weight and stay satisfied.

You must also be sure to drink plenty of water as you switch to a high fiber diet. Remember that fiber tends to retain water. This is good, because it helps to lubricate waste matter as it passes through the intestine. But it also means that your intestine will be able to extract less water from the food you eat than it normally does. So make an effort to drink several glasses of water a day to make up for the deficit.

Water promises many other benefits for the dieter. The most obvious is that it takes up plenty of room in the stomach, and this helps to depress hunger (although those folks who've tried the "water diet" have discovered it can't do the job all by itself!) But water plays hundreds of other roles in good health. The human body is more than 90 percent water, and metabolic processes require water for proper function. Water is not just a low-cal substitute for soda pop; it is the very substance of life. Drink it every chance you get. I Try to find water without chlorine or chemicals in it. It tastes better and is much better for you.

Not everybody can get all the fiber they need strictly from diet, however. In our fast-paced world, you may simply not have the time to munch your way through a pile of celery or apples. Luckily, there are a number of high-fiber supplements you can use to increase your fiber consumption easily. The first of these is a pure cellulose preparation. This is the fiber from plant cell walls, refined and usually offered in pill or tablet form. You take it before meals; it swells in your stomach and acts as a hunger depressant. Now, there's nothing wrong with cellulose *per se*, but I do hesitate to recommend cellulose tablets. First off, they're terribly expensive. Secondly, cellulose itself contains no nutrients other than fiber. I thing there are cheaper, more nutritious ways to get more fiber in your diet. Thirdly, refined cellulose has been shown to be not as effective as other fiber sources in speeding the passage of waste material and increasing fat excretion.[7]

The most traditional fiber supplement is wheat bran. Bran is the seven outer layers of the wheat berry, and it's usually removed by millers in the production of white flour. Wheat bran has a lot going for it. It's very high in fiber—about 44 percent, as compared to about 1 percent for a whole apple. It's also high in other nutrients. One hundred grams contain 16 grams of protein (more than most meat), 1,276 milligrams of phosphorus, 14.9 grams of iron (far more iron than beef liver) and 21 milligrams of niacin and substantial amounts of many other vitamins and minerals.[8] It blends easily with many foods. And, best of all, it's cheap. You can buy a pound of miller's bran for less than a dollar at most health food stores.

However, wheat bran also has a few drawbacks you should be aware of. It has an unusual taste and smell which remind some people of straw.

As a result, you'll normally have to blend the bran with other foods. Also, bran has a very fibrous texture, and has a mouth-feel that some people find disagreeable at first. But many people have reported that they do eventually get used to bran and are able to fit it into their diet comfortably.

Be careful when you buy bran. Many natural food companies are coming out with a finely ground bran, which resembles a brown powder. This has the advantage of blending more invisibly into foods than does coarse miller's bran. But studies have shown that fine bran is far less effective than coarse bran in promoting fat excretion and speeding food through the digestive tract.[9] Plus, fine bran is usually far more expensive than miller's bran, because it requires more processing. So if you're going to use bran as a fiber supplement, it's always wisest to use good old miller's bran.

I myself have developed a high-fiber formula which I feel overcomes many of the problems associated with wheat bran. I mix miller's bran with wheat germ (another high-fiber, high-nutrient residual from the white flour process). I add barley malt, cinnamon and vanilla for flavoring and lecithin for added lubrication and a more pleasing texture. I call the formula FIBRAN, and I market it through Natural Ovens of Manitowoc, Wisconsin. I've included the formula for FIBRAN at the back of this book, in case you'd rather make it yourself.

FIBRAN has many qualities simple wheat

bran can't match. It's got more protein, and is richer in some of the B complex vitamins than bran alone. Its taste and smell are far more pleasing—some folks even like it all by itself, with a little milk and fruit, as a breakfast cereal. The added lecithin gives it a more pleasing mouth-feel, and also adds its own nutritional plus. Lecithin is a good source of choline, and also helps dissolve fat deposits in arteries. I think it's well worth your while to give FIBRAN a try!

Whichever type of fiber supplement you use, you're sure to start reaping the benefits of a high-fiber, high-nutrient, all natural diet immediately. You'll eat to satisfaction, lose weight, and feel better than ever. So why wait a minute longer? Get out there and *eat natural!*

A NOTE ABOUT FIBER

Scientists are still not sure how to determine the amount of fiber in foods. The earliest and most widely-used method was to treat food with acids, alkali, water, alcohol and ether. Anything that could stand up to that kind of rough treatment would easily survive a trip through the digestive system, researchers reasoned. The material left over from this five-solvent process is called crude fiber.

Only recently have nutritionists discovered that crude fiber is not the whole story. Many types of fibers, such as gums, mucilages, pectins and storage polysaccharides, no not survive the crude fiber analytical process, but do play an important part in nutrition. These are called the

SOLUBLE fibers. Soluble fibers don't increase fecal bulk the way insoluble fibers like cellulose, hemicelluloses and lignin do. Instead they retain water and form gels in the intestine which slow the absorption of nutrients across the intestine. This is especially important in the case of carbohydrate absorption; the soluble fibers tend to regulate the passage of simple carbohydrates into the blood stream, thus helping to prevent abnormally high or low blood sugar. Soluble fibers also lower serum cholesterol levels. This kind of fiber decreases low-density lipoproteins (a harmful substance in the blood) and increase the amount of beneficial high-density lipoproteins.

Soluble fibers are an important part of a food's fiber package; in some foods soluble fiber makes up more than 50 percent of the total fiber content. Dietary fiber levels may be as much as 35 times higher than crude fiber figures indicate. Little wonder, then, that recent international conferences on dietary fiber have called for the abandonment of crude fiber listings. As pioneering fiber researcher Dr. Denis Burkitt wrote me, "crude fiber figures. . .are utterly and absolutely meaningless, and ought to be totally abandoned."[10] Consequently, we've decided to drop the crude fiber listings from the first edition and replace them with more complete dietary fiber listing.

Unfortunately, dietary fiber figures are more expensive and time-consuming to obtain than crude fiber values, so it is as yet not possible to present a comprehensive list. The figures we present here have been adapted from those found in a 1978 review published in *Diabetes Care*.[11] Other figures (those without soluble fiber listings) were taken from Paul and Southgate's *The Composition Of Foods*[12]. I have judged them the best available, at least until a more universally-accepted testing method comes along.

Once again, I recommend a daily intake of 50 grams of dietary fiber from all sources.

FIBER LISTINGS

Vegetables—Composition per 100 gm. edible portion.

Item	Total Fiber (gm)	Soluble Fiber (gm)
Asparagus	1.7	.5
Beans, baked	7.3	—
Beans, sprouted	1.8	.6
Beans, string	3.4	1.2
Beets	2.5	1.0
Broccoli	4.1	2.6
Brussels sprouts	2.9	1.2
Cabbage	2.8	1.7
Carrots	3.7	2.5
Cauliflower	1.8	.5
Celery	3.0	.8
Cucumber	1.5	.9
Eggplant	1.5	.9
Endive	2.2	—
Kale greens	3.7	1.5
Leeks	3.9	—
Lentils	3.7	—
Lettuce	1.5	.6
Mushrooms	2.5	—
Onions	2.1	1.0
Parsley	9.1	—
Peppers, green	.9	—
Radishes	2.2	.5
Rutabaga	2.4	1.1
Spinach	6.3	—

Squash, summer	3.0	1.4
Tomatoes	1.4	.4
Turnips	2.2	1.0
Watercress	3.3	—
Zucchini	3.0	1.4

FRUITS

Composition per 100 gm. edible portion.

Item	Total Fiber (gm)	Soluble Fiber (gm)
Apples	3.4	2.0
Apricots	1.7	1.0
Banana	1.8	.9
Blackberries	5.0	.9
Cherries	1.2	.4
Cranberries	4.2	—
Currants, black	8.7	—
Dates	8.7	—
Figs, dried	18.5	—
Grapefruit	1.3	.9
Grapes	.8	.2
Lemons	5.2	—
Muskmelon	1.2	.3
Nectarines	2.4	—
Olives	4.4	—
Orange	2.1	1.6
Peaches	1.3	.7
Pears	2.4	.6
Pineapple	1.0	.3
Plums	1.8	1.0
Prunes, stewed	8.1	—

Raisins	6.8	—
Strawberries	2.1	.8
Tangerines	2.1	1.6

BREADS, CEREAL PRODUCTS AND STARCHY VEGETABLES

Composition per 100 gm. edible portion.

Item	Total Fiber (gm)	Soluble Fiber (gm)
Barley, pearl, boiled	2.2	—
Beans, white	4.7	.5
Beans, kidney	4.8	.5
Beans, pinto	10.0	1.0
Beans, brown	9.7	1.0
Beans, lima	3.7	.4
Bran, 100% cereal	33.1	.9
Bran, wheat	44.0	—
Bread, French	2.9	.1
Bread, rye	10.8	.3
Bread, white	2.7	.1
Bread, whole grain wheat	9.5	.3
Corn, kernels	4.7	1.4
Corn, grits	10.6	3.3
Corn bread	3.4	1.1
Corn flakes	11.0	3.4
Crackers, butter	2.8	.1
Crackers, graham	10.1	.3
Crackers, saltine	3.9	.1
Farina	3.1	.1
Noodles, egg	3.0	.1
Oats, whole	9.0	3.0

Pancakes	1.4	.04
Parsnips	4.9	.5
Peas	7.8	3.0
Popcorn	15.5	4.6
Potatoes, white	3.5	2.0
Rice, brown	5.5	0.0
Rice, white	2.1	0.0
Roll, dinner	2.8	.1
Rye flour, dark	13.9	.4
Rye wafers	11.7	.3
Spaghetti	3.6	.1
Squash, winter	3.5	.4
Sweet Potatoes	4.0	2.2
Waffle	1.5	.05
Wheat flour, whole grain	9.5	.3
Wheat flour, white	3.2	.1
Wheat cereal, flakes	13.1	.4
Wheat cereal, shredded	12.2	.4

NOTES

[1] David Reuben, *The Save Your Life Diet* (New York: Ballantine Books, 1976), p 100.

[2] Reuben, p 102.

[3] A. Antonis et. al., "The Influence of Diet on Fecal Lipids in South African White and Bantu Prisoners," *American Journal of Clinical Nutrition,* Vol. 11, August 1962, pp 142 - 155.

[4] Ray Hill, *Bran* (Wellingborough, Northamptonshire, England: Thorsons Publishers Limited, 1976), p 33.

[5] Peter J. Van Soest, "Some Factors Influencing the Ecology of Gut Fermentation in Man," *Gastrointestinal Cancer: Endogenous Factors* (Cold Spring Harbor Laboratory, 1981).

[6] Bonnie Liebman, "Facts About Fiber," *Nutrition Action,* March 1982, p 17.

[7] Van Soest, ibid.

[8] United States Department of Agriculture, *Composition of Foods* (Washington, D.C.: U.S. Govt. Printing Office, 1975), p 66.

[9] Van Soest, op. cit.

[10] Denis Burkitt, personal correspondence, February 17, 1982.

[11] James W. Anderson, Wen-Ju Lin and Kyleen Ward, "Composition of Foods Commonly Used in Diets for Persons with Diabetes," *Diabetes Care,* Vol. 1 No. 5, September-October 1978, pp 296 - 298.

[12] A.A. Paul and D.A.T. Southgate, *The Composition of Foods* (New York: Elsevier/North-Holland Biomedical Press).

6

FOOD ADDICTIONS:
They can make you fat — and drive you crazy!

Is there one food you really love? I'm not talking about some once-in-a-while treat you find pleasurable. I'm talking about the foods you're crazy for, foods you eat every day, foods you binge on.

Do you have a food like this, a food you KNOW is good for you?

Then get rid of it!

A passionate love affair with any food—be it milk, wheat, corn, sugar or anything else—is a good sign that you may be *addicted* to it. That addiction can be causing you to overeat, and distort your metabolism so that weight-loss becomes almost impossible.

The phenomenon of food addiction is one of the most puzzling and frustrating experiences a dieter can face. The food addict must be constantly exposed to the food to which he or she is addicted; the alternative can be headache, depression, lethargy or even unconsciousness—all classic withdrawal symptoms.

And, despite the fact that the substance to which one is addicted is a food, the food addict often shows the same types of dependencies seen in drug addicts. According to Dr. Richard MacKarness, "In my opinion, only heroin or morphine addiction is more potent and destructive than severe food addiction, which I would put on a par with alcoholism."[1]

What *is* a food addiction? What causes it? How can you detect it? And how can you get rid of it?

Actually, a food addiction is physiologically very similar to other types of addictions. All foods contain minor irritants—you might call them mild poisons—that are unique to them. If you eat a food only occasionally—say, once a week—these toxins are eliminated from the body and cause no harm. But the components of the average American diet have become so limited that there are many foods and food ingredients that we eat every day, or even every meal. For instance, the average American eats 120 pounds of wheat flour every year, but only 10 pounds of rice. Each American eats over 100 pounds of beef and veal, but only 45 pounds of chicken, 10 pounds each of turkey and organ meats, 1 pound of lamb and mutton and less than a pound of duck and goose each year. We consume twice as much processed citrus foods (primarily orange juice) than similar non-citrus items.[2] Because we eat these foods so frequently, their specific toxins build up in the body, and cause a negative reaction.

The body has a remarkable way of adjusting to the stress caused by constant exposure to these toxins. Eventually the body's biochemistry changes to take account for the toxin; when this happens, the toxin actually becomes a "needed" substance. Abstinence from the food for even a few hours can cause depressive withdrawal symptoms, which disappear when the individual eats the food again. The person may even feel high, happy and self-confident after being re-exposed to the food toxin, much in the way that a heroin addict feels high after getting a fix of his favorite toxin. This transformation of a food substance from a poison to a "need" is called a *maladaptive reaction.*[3]

Because the formation of a maladaptive reaction requires a build-up of the toxin in the body, it follows that the foods you eat most often are the ones you stand the greatest chance of forming an addiction to. In my opinion, the most addictive substances Americans deal with are sugar, caffeine, alcohol, chocolate, wheat, corn, milk, egg, potato and orange. Other addictive substances that wreak havoc on diet are cigarettes, tranquilizers, uppers and illegal drugs.

Most of us have no idea if we've formed maladaptive reactions, because we structure our lives so that we are never long without our fix. If you're allergic to milk, for instance, you may have a glass of milk at every meal and another glass at bedtime; a cheese sandwich for lunch or cheese as an evening snack; cream in every cup of coffee. You may even wake up in the middle of the night, unable to get back to sleep until you've had a glass of warm milk. No one thinks this is odd behavior—in fact, it's the kind of thing the

American Dairy Association's been trying to get you to do for years!

But the truth is that your constant consumption of milk is fueled by an addiction: if you get your milk fix, you feel fine, and if you don't, you get sick.

Yet even though you feel OK by constantly exposing yourself to the food you're addicted to, all is not well. Try as it might, your body cannot compensate entirely for the presence of the toxins in these foods. The metabolic shock they create interferes with pancreatic function, thus contributing to hypoglycemia, intestinal acidosis and disturbed fat metabolism. These things in turn increase the body's sensitivity to toxins—and the cycle continues again. Some doctors believe that all human degenerative diseases can be traced to the physical punishment caused by this addiction cycle.[4] Food addictions can also cause adrenal exhuastion. It is known that people trapped in a food addiction cycle sometimes suffer from asthma, itching, depression, arthritis, chest pains, rapid or irregular pulse, hypertension, anemia, lethargy, paranoia and even coma.[5]

Although the punishment of a food addiction can damage every system in the body, we are especially concerned here with how it affects your weight. Food addiction can be a nightmare for dieters for two reasons. In the first place, the food addict has no control over his or her food intake. The addict *must* consume the addictive food, often in truly amazing amounts, or risk withdrawal pains. Frequently addicts go on a binge in which they cannot stop themselves from wolfing down huge quantities of their favorite food. Such a food dependency adds enormous amounts of food energy to the diet— food energy that is converted into fat.

Let's look at one example—the example of milk addiction. Some researchers estimate that as many as 40 percent of all Americans may have a maladaptive reaction to milk and milk products. A milk addict may consume up to 113 ounces of milk or more *a day*—not counting cream, cheese, cottage cheese or ice cream.[6] That adds up to more than 2,200 calories daily— calories that are consumed, not because the body needs or can use that much food energy, but as the result of a destructive addiction.

Secondly, maladaptive reactions can severely distort the body's metabolism. Maladaptive reactions can cause pancreatic malfunction, leading to acute acidosis in the small intestine (thus disrupting amino acid metabolism) and lowered lipase activity (which hinders the body's metabolism of fats). These changes can prevent your body from getting rid of excess fat—no matter how stringently you diet and how hard you exercise. I know—I once had a small "spare tire" around my midsection which refused to go away, despite a natural foods diet and plenty of exercise. But when I discovered and got rid of my food allergies, the stubborn fat left in a matter of days! I was able to metabolize the fat. All other people should pray for more enzymes to break down their fat.

Food addictions have drawn the most attention because of their psychological aspects—depression, neurosis, even schizophrenia. But I believe that understanding the phenomenon of maladaptive reactions is of tremendous importance to those who are trying to lose weight as well.

The benefits of freeing yourself from food addictions can be tremendous. Dr. Theron Randolph, pioneer in the study of food addictions, notes the case of a middle-aged woman whose problems went far beyond obesity; she had required hospitalization for depression, had attempted suicide twice and had been given electroshock therapy. It was discovered that the woman had an addiction to peanuts, yeast and milk—three primary ingredients of the peanut butter sandwich, a food she had eaten addictively for years. When she avoided these foods—and broke out of the addictive cycle—not only did her psychiatric problems clear up, but she also lost a significant amount of weight.[7]

Dr. Arthur Coca has had similar success in treating obesity by detecting and reversing food addiction. "Miss M.," age 50, was only moderately overweight at 140 pounds, but she felt the added weight was an annoying encumberance. She also suffered migraine headaches, tiredness, constipation, occasional dizziness and sinusitis. She ate a broad range of reactive foods: cow's milk, cereals, all meats but pork, citrus fruits and cane sugar. She avoided these substances and lost more than 10 pounds in four weeks.

"Of course she lost weight," you might say to yourself, "there was nothing left for her to eat!" In fact, nothing could be further from the truth. As Dr. Coca reports, "There was not any starvation; Miss M. never felt hungry, as she often had when she was fat. She ate to her appetite's content of her many safe foods including potato, sweet potato, dates, peas, beans. . ."

Dr. Coca also reports the case of Mrs. B, who lost 35 pounds with a diet which did *not* restrict carbohydrates, and which let her eat as much as she wanted of non-addictive foods. She only had to avoid cow's milk, citrus fruit, carrots, beet greens, asparagus, onion and nuts.[8]

How do you find out what kinds of food addictions you have, and how do you correct them?

Doctors have two ways of detecting maladaptive reactions. Both involve clearing the body of built-up toxins, and then testing suspect foods one at a time. After the body has been cleared of toxins, it becomes hypersensitive to them, so that their reintroduction can cause symptoms far more noticeable than those the individual suffered when eating the food every day.

One way to clear the body of toxins is to go on a four-day fast, in which only distilled or spring water is consumed. In this way the body's exposure to toxins is completely eliminated, and the metabolism is given the opportunity to return to normal. Many doctors prefer this method, primarily because it is simple and fast, but I don't recommend that you try it without medical supervision. In the first place, the withdrawal symptoms you may suffer can be quite intense, and it may be risky to try to handle them on your own. Secondly, if you are diabetic, pre-diabetic or severely hypoglycemic (many people are and don't suspect it), it could be positively dangerous for you to go without any source of food for four days. Fasting can be a great experience for people in good health—but the obese individual is by definition unhealthy.

The other alternative is to use a rotation diet. In this diet, no food is eaten more frequently than once every four days, and certain of the "worst offender" foods are eliminated entirely. The idea here is to keep the levels of various toxins so low and infrequent that the body has time to clear itself. The advantage to this approach is that it allows you to *eat* (with a lot more variety than you've probably ever experienced), and so is less stressful to the body than a spring water fast. You must allow more time for the body to correct itself, however, and that is one drawback.

Some rotation diets can be awfully complex, but a few simple—and effective—diets do exist. The one I present here has been adapted from *The Supernutrition Handbook,* by Patrick Mooney.[9] I strongly recommend that you try to identify your hidden food addictions using this rotation diet at the outset of your weight loss program; neglecting to do so could sabotage your efforts to trim down, for reasons we've already discussed.

The first step in using this rotation diet is to identify suspected foods to which you might be addicted. Information gained from filling out the Body Wisdom Diary can be very helpful in doing this. Note especially foods that you really love to eat and that you consume frequently. All such foods should be suspect—and will be tested after clearing the body of the toxins in these foods. In addition, if you notice that these foods make you feel "high" immediately after you've eaten them, but are accompanied by negative symptoms several hours later, this is a very strong indication that you are addicted.

The next step is to actually begin the rotation diet. It consists of a four-day cycle, which you repeat twice. You may eat as much as you like of the foods that are allowed for that day. Many prime addictive foods are already eliminated from this diet; you should also eliminate listed foods which you suspect you may be addicted to.

Be careful of prepared foods, like bread, during this phase of the diet, because its ingredients are in several different groups. For example, a normal bread may contain wheat, sugar, corn, barley, soybean oil, cottonseed oil, oat flour, yeast and possibly a host of chemicals used for flavoring, coloring or preserving. For this part of the diet it's best that you eat only simple, unprocessed foods.

Here's the diet itself. You might find it convenient to take it with you when you shop.

DAY ONE

PROTEIN:
  Lamb
  Rabbit Family
  Salmon/Trout Family
  Whitefish Family
  Catfish Family
  Sea Bass Family
  (Grouper, Rockfish,
  Sea Basses, White Perch)

SPROUTS:
  Sunflower Seed Sprouts

GREENS:
  Endive
  Escarole
  Artichoke
  Dandelion
  Lily Family
  (Asparagus, Chives, Leek Greens, Yucca)

LEGUMES:
  Sweet Potato Family
  Water Chestnut Family

VEGGIES:
  Yam Family
  Avacado

NUTS & SEEDS:
  Sunflower Seeds
  Hazelnut Family
  (Hazelnuts, Filberts)

FRUITS:
  Rose Family
  (Pear, Strawberry, Blackberry, Raspberry)

SPICES:
  Safflower
  Chicory
  Goldenrod
  Nutmeg Family
  (Nutmeg, Mace)
  Sassafras

DAY TWO

PROTEIN:
  Grass Family
  (Barley, Oats, Millet, Rice)

SPROUTS:
  Legume Family
  (Lentil Sprouts, Alfalfa Sprouts)

GREENS:
  Carrot Family
  (Parsley, Celery Greens)

LEGUMES:
  Carrot Family
  Carrots, Celery,

VEGGIES:
  Parsnips
  Legume Family
  (Lentils, Alfalfa, Peas)
  Mushroom Family

NUTS & SEEDS:
  Hickory Nut Family
  Chestnut Family
  Litchi Nut Family

FRUITS:
  Pineapple Family
  Persimmon Family

SPICES:
  Legume Family
  (Carob, Gum Acacia, Lecithin)
  Palm Family
  (Coconut, Sage, Date Palm, Sago)
  Vanilla Family

DAY THREE

PROTEIN:
  Chicken Family
  (Quail, Cornish Hen, Pheasant, Peafowl)
  Turkey Family
  Duck Family
  Goose Family

GREENS:
  Mustard Family
  (Collards, Broccoli, Brussels Sprouts, Kale

Turnip Greens, Cabbage, Mustard Greens)

LEGUMES:
  Mustard Family
  Horseradish, Mustard

VEGGIES:
  Rutabaga, Turnips
  Cauliflower, Bok Choy

NUTS & SEEDS:
  Cashew Family
  (Pistachios)
  Sesame Seed Family
  Flax Seed Family

FRUITS:
  Cashew Family
  (Mangos)
  Papaya Family
SPICES:
  Mint Family
  (Peppermint, Basil, Spearmint, Sage,
  Marjoram, Savory, Horehound, Thyme,
  Rosemary, Lavender, Chinese Artichoke)

DAY FOUR
PROTEIN:
  Sole Family
  Mackeral Family
  (Jack Mackeral, Pompano)
  Flounder/Halibut Family

Freshwater Bass Family
(Sunfish, Bluegills, Basses)

GREENS:
Beet Family
(Beets, Spinach, Swiss Chard)

LEGUMES:
Squash Family
(Squashes, Zucchini)

VEGGIES:
Eggplant

NUTS & SEEDS:
Squash Family
(Pumpkin Seeds)
Macadamia Nut Family

FRUITS:
Squash Family
(Honeydew, Muskmelon, Casaba,
Watermelon, Cantelope)

SPICES:
Ginger Family
(Ginger, Tumeric)
Myrtle Family
(Guava, Allspice)

To help you follow the rotation diet, we will give one example of how you could plan meals which would follow the rotation plan:

DAY ONE
SAMPLE BREAKFAST
Diced pears and/or Strawberries with sunflower sees on top, sassafrass tea.
SAMPLE LUNCH
Broiled Whitefish.

Asparagus

Endive, dandelion salad

SAMPLE SUPPER
Salmon or trout—broiled (no butter or lemon)

Baked yams

Avocado, endive, escarole salad with sprouted sunflower seeds.

Fresh or frozen strawberries or pears for dessert. Eat all you want at each meal. Between meal snacks: raw sunflower seeds or filberts.

DAY TWO
SAMPLE BREAKFAST
Rolled barley or oats or millet

(3 oz. grain to 9 oz. water)

Fresh pineapple slices

SAMPLE LUNCH
Soup (combine lentils, carrots, peas, celery, alfalfa sprouts, rice and mushrooms)

Persimmon for dessert.

SAMPLE SUPPER
   Steam some of the vegetables listed above
   Make salad of carrots, celery greens and parsnips
   Persimmon or pineapple for dessert
   Eat all you want at each meal. Between meal snacks: coconut, hickory nuts or chestnuts.

DAY THREE
SAMPLE BREAKFAST
   ½ cornish hen (baked)
   Fresh papaya or mango fruit

SAMPLE LUNCH
   Other ½ cornish hen or turkey
   Steamed rutabaga or turnips with greens
   Broccoli
   Papaya or mango for dessert, with sesame seeds sprinkled over.

SAMPLE SUPPER
   Raw cashews—dry roast them yourself (no oil)
   Steamed cabbage
   Turkey or cornish hen
   Papaya or mango for dessert
   Eat all you want at each meal. Between meal snacks: cashews or pistachio nuts

DAY FOUR
SAMPLE BREAKFAST
Honeydew melon or cantaloupe with raw pumpkin seeds or macadamia nuts
Baked sole or bass if desired

SAMPLE LUNCH
Any of the fish—baked or boiled (no butter)
Baked squash (butternut is excellent)
Beets w/greens (boiled or steamed)
Watermelon for dessert

SAMPLE SUPPER:
Any of the fish
Spinach
Zucchini or squash
Any of the melons listed as dessert. Eat all you want at any meal. Between meal snacks: pumpkin seeds (raw) or macadamia nuts.

Continue this cycle twice, so that you are on the diet for eight days. As your body clears itself of toxins, you'll probably begin to experience some withdrawal symptoms—headache, cravings, depression, etc. After about the third or fourth days, however, these ought to clear up, and you'll really begin to feel great—free at last of all those symptoms you used to think were "normal." Even better, you'll be the master of those addictive foods, instead of their slave.

After eight days on the rotation diet, you begin to reintroduce the eliminated foods, and start filling out the Body Wisdom Diary in Chapter 10.

These include the sources of sugars (beet, cane and corn), alcohol, caffeine, wheat and other grains, milk products, yeast, beef, eggs, chocolate, high-sugar fruits, and, of course, all the foods you've noticed that produced negative reactions in the past. Continue on the foods listed in the rotation diet, and introduce one new food at each meal, and wait for up to three hours for symptoms to appear. If they do not, then you are probably not sensitive to that food. If symptoms DO appear, however, you know that that food was a source of addiction, and you should eliminate it from your diet, at least for 90 days. Also, you ought to wait for the symptoms to go away before you test a new food.

One word about the negative symptoms which can appear from the foods you test: they can be quite severe. They may range from a fit of sneezing to a schizophrenic episode or even a blackout. This is why it may be a good idea to let your doctor know you're going on the rotation diet, *especially if you have a history of depression and other mental illness or severe physical illness.* If a negative reaction becomes extremely uncomfortable, they can usually be eliminated by taking 1,000 to 6,000 mg. of vitamin C, 1,000 mg. of B3, 200 mg. of B6, 250 mg. of B1 and 1 mg of folic acid.[10] These will help the body fight off the negative effects of the toxins.
the negative effects of the toxins.

When you discover that you have a negative reaction to a food, eliminate it from your diet for at least 90 days. This may give the body time to "desensitize" itself to the toxin. After 90 days, eat the food every day for three days and watch for symptoms. If none appear, it means you have become desensitized to the food, and may eat it again *in moderation* (ie., probably no more than once every four days). If symptoms still develop after 90 days, it's best that you never eat that food again.

How do you avoid forming new addictions? The best way is to never eat a food too frequently. It's probably not necessary to maintain the elaborate scheme found in the rotation diet, but if you're eating some food substance more than once a day, every day of the week, you may be creating a risk. The Miracle Menu Plan, included at the end of this book, is designed to give you high nutritional density and high fiber, with enough variety so that the danger of food addiction is minimized.

Another way to prevent the formation of new addictions is to supplement your diet with extra vitamin C (1,000 to 6,000 daily or more, depending on your personal need) and 50 to 200-mg of a high-potency B-complex supplement.

Like other aspects of dieting, relieving yourself of food addictions will have a tremendous impact on your entire life. But best of all, getting free of food addictions may be the most important first step in losing the weight you've always wanted to lose, but never could somehow. Few have put it as simply as Dr. Arthur Coca: "Discover what thing or things are causing your body to retain the extra weight. Avoid them. And watch the pounds go by." [11]

NOTES

[1] Richard MacKarness, "'But I Like It,' The Hazards of Hidden Allergies," *The Health Quarterly,* Vol. 1 No. 4, pp. 44-45, 76, 93.

[2] Letita Brewster and Michael F. Jacobsen, *The Changing American Diet* (Washington, DC: Center for Science in the Public Interest, 1978).

[3] William H. Philpott and Dwight K. Kalita, *Brain Allergies* (New Canaan, Connecticut: Keats Publishing, Inc., 1980), pp. 23-25.

[4] Philpott and Kalita, *Brain Allergies,* p. 103.

[5] Theron G. Randolph and Ralph W. Moss, *An Alternative Approach To Allergies* (New York: Lippincott & Crowell, Publishers, 1980), p. 30.

[6] Alexander Schauss, *Diet Crime and Delinquency* (Berkeley, California: Parker House, 1981), p. 14.

[7] Randolph and Moss, *An Alternative Approach To Allergies,* pp. 151-152

[8] Arthur F. Coca, *The Pulse Test* (New York: Lyle Stuart, 1967), pp. 84-88.

[9] Patrick Mooney, *The Supernutrition Handbook* (Self-published, 1978), pp. 89-109.

[10] Philpott and Kalita, *Brain Allergies,* p. 52.

[11] Coca, *The Pulse Test,* p. 88.

7

WHOLE GRAINS
The Perfect Diet Food

"I'd love to eat more whole wheat bread, but I'm on a diet."

I wish you could see how my teeth grind every time someone says that to me. People have gotten the idea that grain foods—especially bread—are monstrously fattening. So they turn to food that they think is less fattening: meat, vegetables, or one of the preposterous "diet foods," which are nothing but nutritional disasters propped up with all sorts of artificial flavors and colors and every imaginable chemical additive.

In reality, whole grain foods are the *perfect* diet food. They're high in fiber, low in fat, provide a good source of protein, and supply the complex carbohydrates your body needs. And, best of all, whole grain foods are *satisfying*.

Let's look at the facts:

Obesity has become an enormous problem in the United States at the same time Americans are eating less foods made from grain. In 1910, the average American ate about 300 pounds of flour and cereal products. At the same time, grain foods were our *primary* source of protein. Today, however, our consumption of grain is down to 150 pounds a year—most of it in the form of nutritionally denuded white flour products![1]

And what has taken the place of grain foods in the American diet? Meat consumption is up 50 percent since 1930, sugar consumption is up more than 2,500 percent since the turn of the century, and consumption of fat, candy, soft drinks and caffeine is up considerably as well![2] *These* are the foods that are making us fat. It was by turning *away* from grain foods that we took the first step down the road to epidemic obesity.

Our modern diet is so hopelessly out of whack that even the Government is worried. In January 1977, the Senate Select Committee on Nutrition and Human Needs published a study which expressed alarm at current American dietary patterns and called for radical changes in the way we eat. Among its recommendations was that we increase our consumption of complex carbohydrates (the kind provided by bread and other grain foods) from 28 percent of total calories to 48 percent, while we cut our consumption of fat from 40 percent to 30 percent of total energy intake![3] What's the best way to do all this? By simply replacing the meat in our diet with whole grains.

As nutrition expert Michael Jacobson notes, "Bread used to be the staff of life, providing a large percentage of our caloric and nutrient intake. In some cultures, rice, bread or pasta remains the main course for most people. *It is in this direction that we should try to move.* Doing so means eating more slices of bread in the morning to replace an egg. For lunch it means an extra sandwich and no soda pop. For dinner, the beef stroganoff should be heavy on the noodles, using the beef more as a condiment than the main attraction" (emphasis mine).[4] I can only add that this is the perfect prescription for dieters.

Still you're hesitant. Probably all your life you've thought of grain foods, and indeed all carbohydrate foods, as inherently fattening. The whole idea behind the revolutionary "Low-Carbohydrate" diet was that carbohydrates are the most fattening things you could eat. As long as you avoided them, you'd lose weight, no matter what else you ate (so the story went). If these thoughts still trouble you, you need to understand the misconceptions behind the Great Carbohydrate Hoax.

The Hoax begins with the observation that carbohydrates are the body's primary source of energy. This is true. Carbohydrates are molecules made up of carbon, hydrogen and oxygen. They are broken down into glucose, or blood sugar, and glucose is turned to pyruvate to fuel the citric acid cycle, which is the metabolic process that creates all our energy. Other substances, such as amino acids from protein and glycerol and fatty acids from fat can be used to fuel the cycle, but glucose is the body's favorite fuel.

Now, this is how the Hoax proceeds. By eating

carbohydrates, we provide our bodies with a lot of readily available glucose, which is turned into energy—too much energy. The excess energy is turned in to fat, and that we don't want. So (says the Hoax), the thing to do is stop eating carbohydrates and fill up on something else— protein is usually the "something," although fat is also sometimes suggested. Thus we deprive ourselves of carbohydrates, reduce the glucose in the blood, cut of the body's favorite energy food and voila! No more excess energy, no more ugly fat!

But here's where the Hoax runs against the great unwritten law of biochemistry: Your body isn't as dumb as the experts think. Sure, it prefers to make energy out of carbohydrates, but it's extremely adaptable. When the diet is low in carbohydrates but high in protein or fat, your metabolism can shift from a reliance on glucose to a reliance on fatty or amino acids. Your body isn't fooled. You don't deprive your body of energy by stuffing yourself with protein instead of carbohydrates.

In fact, there's an irony in the Great Carbohydrate Hoax. In order to cut down on carbohydrates and turn on to protein, dieters eat a lot of meat. But while meat may contain protein, it contains a lot more fat. A pound of choice sirloin, for instance, may contain 71.1 grams of protein, but it also has 112.3 grams of fat.[5] Ham contains about twice as much fat as protein.[6] Even chicken and fish contain about a third as much fat as protein. The upshot is, a high-meat diet is a high-fat diet. And fat releases twice as much food energy as carbohydrate. So for some people a low-carbohydrated diet may be more fattening than a high-carbohydrate diet.

Not only is a high-protein, low-carbohydrate diet ineffective for healthy, long-term weight loss; it can be extremely dangerous. We said that the body can use glucose, amino acids or fatty acids for energy. There's one crucial exception: the brain. Due to the unique characteristics of the blood-brain berrier, the brain can use only glucose for fuel. Although the liver can synthesize some glucose from protein, there's no doubt that a low-carbohydrate diet means lowered blood sugar—hypoglycemia. Robbed of glucose, the delicate tissues of the brain are the first to suffer.

Taking the high-protein path to avoid carbohydrates has other hazardous side-effects, and we'll deal with them in Chapter 9. It is enough to say here that the human body simply isn't set up to handle excessive protein. This makes sense, given our vegetarian ancestry. But the modern dieter who turns to protein as an alternative to "fattening" carbohydrates is setting him- or herself up for disaster.

We have established that our bodies need carbohydrates to survive, and that a low-carbohydrate regimen is not a safe path to weight loss. But there are lots of different kinds of carbohydrates, and dieters must choose the right ones.

The best carbohydrates for dieters are the *complex carbohydrates*. You know them as

starches. We've already talked about some of the
dangers associated with simple carbohydrates,
especially sucrose: besides being potent appetite
stimulants, simple carbohydrates are addictive.
They tend to enter the bloodstream very quickly
and all at once, and so engender a metabolic
overreaction which leads to hypoglycemia. We've
mentioned this as a reason for avoiding sugar
(and the processed foods containing sugar), but
at the same time it's also a good reason for the
dieter to turn to complex carbohydrates. Because
they are indeed chemically more complex (they
are actually long, entangled strings of simpler
sugars), they enter the bloodstream more slowly,
and don't foster the low blood sugar which
causes ravenous hunger. They don't have a
damaging hit-and-run effect, as simple sugar
does.

That's what your mother meant when she said
that a high-starch food like old fashioned
oatmeal "sticks to your ribs." Complex
carbohydrates are satisfying carbohydrates.

Researchers in Canada have demonstrated
the superiority of complex carbohydrates as an
aid to weight loss. In 1973 a study at the
University of Guelph, doctors fed rats diets
which contained equivalent amounts of
carbohydrate. However, some rats got their
carbohydrate from sucrose, while others got
theirs from corn starch.

The rats on the high-sucrose diet showed
significantly faster weight gain and higher body
fat levels than the rats on starch, even though

they all received the same amount of carbohydrate[7]

Similarly, British researchers at Queen Elizabeth College discovered that animals maintained on a sucrose-rich diet had significantly higher plasma tryglyceride concentrations than their litter-mates given starch[8] Since tryglycerides are stored in adipose tissue as fat, this study once again indicates the superiority of complex carbohydrates in a weight loss diet.

And what are the best sources of complex carbohydrates? Ah, at last we come around again to our original point. Whole grains are the richest, most nutritionally balanced source of complex carbohydrates. Wheat is 70 to 70 percent carbohydrate, virtually all of it complex. Barley is 78 percent, oats are 68 percent. These compare very favorably to other vegetable products: Beets are only 9.9 percent carbohydrate, cabbage 5.2 percent, Grapefruit 10.6 percent. Of course, meat and dairy products contain no carbohydrates whatsoever. Ounce for ounce, whole grains deliver more of the complex carbohydrates your body needs than any other food.

Whole grains provide a lot more than just carbohydrates. They are an excellent source of protein. Today we don't think of grains as protein foods, but the fact is that just seventy years ago flour and other cereal products provided about 40 percent of our protein—more protein than meat, dairy products or eggs. Our grandparents relied on vegetable products for half their total protein consumption[9]—and few of them died of any protein deficiency diseases. We simply have to rid ourselves of the notion that protein means meat.

Whole wheat flour is 13.3 percent protein. Some of the special components of wheat are even higher: wheat bran is 16 percent and wheat germ is 26.6 percent. Barley and millet are about 10 percent protein, and rolled oats contain 14 percent. Now, this may not seem like much as compared to 23 percent protein in choice sirloin, but remember the fat factor. Whole wheat bread's protein-to-fat ratio is *five times* higher than sirloin's. Whole grains are a low-fat source of protein, and that is precisely what the dieter needs.

Of course, any single whole grain isn't a protein panacea. Whole wheat flour, for instance, is a bit deficient in the important amino acid lycine, which is why many whole wheat breads are fortified with oat flour, soybean flour, or extra bran or germ, all of which are plentiful in lysine. Eating a variety of whole grains, and supplementing your diet with beans, legumes and moderate amounts of eggs and dairy products will help you be sure you're getting plenty of all essential amino acids. But remember to make whole grains the foundation of your protein picture.

Whole grains are an excellent source of another important nutrient: fiber. We saw in Chapter Five that fiber makes food more satisfying and maintains the efficiency of the digestive tract. Well, whole grains are superior fiber sources for three reasons. They provide the most fiber, they provide the best kind of fiber, and they provide the most efficient form of fiber. Let me explain.

In terms of quantity alone, whole grains have almost all other fiber sources beat cold. Whole wheat flour contains 9.5 percent dietary fiber, oats 9 percent and rye flour 13.9 percent. The only vegetable sources that can match these figures are nuts (which are high in fat) and certain berries and dried fruits (which are high in simple carbohydrates). A single slice of whole grain bread provides 2.7 grams of dietary fiber, more than that provided by a half cup of any vegetable other than peas, parsnips or potatoes.

Furthermore, whole grains give you the best kind of fiber—cellulose. While your body needs all of the dietary fibers, cellulose is the most important in creating a feeling of satiety and moving digested material rapidly through the intestinal tract. The bran layers of whole grains are very high in cellulose—wheat bran being the most notable in this regard. Laboratory studies and clinical tests have so frequently demonstrated the superiority and efficiency of grain fiber in digestive function that Dr. Denis Burkitt maintains "It is essential to emphasize that cereals are a vastly better source of fiber than green vegetables and fruit, and things like celery and salad are little more than packaged water."

Thirdly, whole-grains—especially coarsely-ground whole grains, provide the best *form* of fiber. The shape of bran as it comes off the wheat berry in the stone-grinding process enables it to take up the maximum amount of space in the stomach and in the intestines, and to absorb and retain the most water. Coarse bran has been compared to chemical laxatives, cabbage fiber and even finely ground bran itself. In every instance bran has been found the most effective form of fiber. Whole grains are, quite simply the premier fiber source for the human digestive system.

Complex carbohydrates, protein, fiber—these are things the dieter needs most, and these are the things whole grain foods provide. How can you work more whole grains into your diet? Eating more whole grain bread is an obvious answer, but many of us would be hard-pressed to think of other uses for whole grains.

The good news is there are a lot of ways to get into grains. Cracked wheat cereal and rolled oats are two foods more dieters ought to discover. They make great hot cereals for breakfast, of course. And when cracked wheat is soaked overnight in water (a process which retains the maximum amount of nutrition), it makes the base for tabouli, a tasty salad from the middle east. Cracked wheat can also be used as a filler for meat dishes. Whole wheat can be uses in falafil, a sort of spicy dough-like paste which is rolled into balls or pressed into patties and then fried. Whole wheat pastas are getting easier to find, and whole wheat noodles make a superior lasagna.

Those of you who have formed addictive, maladaptive reactions to a specific grain will have to exercise a little caution and selectivity. Yet there are so many kinds of whole grains that even if you're especially sensitive to wheat, for instance, you can still enjoy buckwheat, brown rice, millet, and many others.

They're delicious, they're nutritious and they're extremely versatile; what more need I say? If you're trying to lose weight, you owe it to yourself to discover whole grains!

NOTES

[1] Letitia Brewster and Michael F. Jacobson, *The Changing American Diet* (Washington, D.C.: Center for Science in the Public Interest, 1978), p. 26.

[2] Brewster and Jacobson, *The Changing American Diet*, p. 4.

[3] Select Committee on Nutrition and Human Needs, United States Senate, *Dietary Goals For The United States* (Washington, D.C.: U.S. Govt. Printing Office, 1977).

* [4] Michael Jacobson, *"Pass The Pasta, Please,"* Shape, March 1982, pp. 83-85.

[5] United States Department of Agriculture, *Composition Of Foods* (Washington, D.C.: U.S. Govt. Printing Office, 1963), p. 15.

[6] USDA, *Composition of Foods*, p. 50.

[7] Research Notes

[8] Research Notes

[9] Brewster and Jacobson, *The Changing American Diet*, p. 65.

8

EXERCISE:
Solving Your Energy Crisis

Well, that's it. You've learned why the traditional calorie-counting diet doesn't work, and you've seen that dieters who try to live on processed foods are doomed to failure. You've learned about the two important factors in the satisfaction equation—nutritional density and fiber— and how they can help you feel full and healthy while you lose weight and keep it off. You've seen how you can escape the slavery of food addictions. Most of all, you've learned that the most effective weight-control diet is a *natural* diet filled with delicious, whole foods.

Now, if I were like most diet writers, I'd stop here. After all, I've shown you how to lower your caloric intake effectively, effortlessly and naturally, without having to "count" anything. But I feel I'd be irresponsible to leave you here, because I realize that *dieting alone is not enough.* What's missing? *Exercise!*

Many people today think it's enough to simply cut down on calories in a weight-loss program. And it's easy to see how they make this mistake.

It has been traditional for doctors and nutritionists to discuss human nutrition in terms of an oversimplified "calorie equation." They point out that people gain weight because they consume too much food energy—too many calories. The solution, they say, is either to cut down on energy intake (by dieting) or increase energy output (by exercise). Some even go to the absurd point of suggesting that if you eat some specific food you must do some specific amount of exercise, as if 100 sit-ups will counteract a forbidden slice of cheesecake! We've already seen that human biochemical individuality insures that such "calorie-swaps" work only in the imagination of diet doctors. More importantly, since many people in our society hate hard physical labor, they opt to cut their energy balance by cutting out calories.

The problem is that, while the calorie equation is technically correct, it is vastly oversimplified. Cutting energy intake through diet and increasing energy output through exercise are not two separate but equal alternatives. In order to lose weight safely, *you must do both.* Here's why.

Your body has two major storage substances, protein and fat. When your energy intake is less than your energy output, your body draws on these two sources of stored calories. Of the two, protein breaks down much more rapidly than fat.

When you diet without exercise, then, your body first turns to its protein stores—which are the body tissues themselves. Muscle tissue especially is broken down and converted to amino acids which are used for energy. The result is muscle degradation and general loss of muscle tone. This accounts for some of the weakness that many dieters feel.

When you diet *and* exercise, though, something called the Training Effect comes into play. When you exercise, your body builds muscle and so uses available amino acids for muscle construction and maintenance. Your body must then turn to its other storage facility, the fat cells, to make up the energy deficit. Thus, when you diet and exercise, your muscle tone is improved and your body fat is consumed. Instead of becoming tired and flabby, you're firm and full of energy. Of course, initially your weight loss may not be terribly fast, because you are gaining muscle weight at the same time you are losing fat weight. In some cases, you may not lose any weight at all for the first few weeks (you will *feel* a lot better, though!) Just keep at it. After the first few weeks, your weight loss will start to show up on the scale.

This is why I always recommend exercise, even though I'm a biochemist and not an exercise expert. I realize that a person MUST exercise if he or she is to remain healthy during weight loss. Exercise is not just a good idea; it's *crucial.*

However, I do stress nutrition over exercise. The reason is that strenuous activity increases the demands your body makes on its metabolism.

If your metabolism has been distorted through nutrient deficiency it cannot meet these increased demands. If you try to exercise on a junk food diet, you'll find that you just don't have the energy to continue. You'll give up. That's why I recommend that you get on a natural foods diet before you begin an exercise program. That way exercise will be an ecstasy, not an agony!

There are a whole galaxy of benefits that come from combining exercise with diet. Most of these spring from the fact that exercise strengthens the cardio-pulmonary and cardio-vascular systems. As you exercise, your heart, lungs, arteries and veins get a workout too. They become more efficient. Circulation improves, and the entire body gets a rich supply of blood. The first benefit to this is that it insures that the nutrients you get from your food are better distributed through the body. Eating foods with a high nutritional density will do you no good if the vitamins and minerals can't get to the parts of the body where they're needed!

A second big benefit from improved circulation is that it supplies more oxygen to the cells. Most of us learned in school that the body uses oxygen to burn fuel for energy. If your circulation remains poor your cells get insufficient oxygen and cannot produce energy effectively. When this happens, *all* of the cell's functions, from respiration to reproduction, are critically impaired, because they all require energy. Simply put, your body malfunctions. Without proper circulation, you cannot tap your body's full potential. *With* proper circulation, you can be the fantastically alive person you were meant to be!

Exercise shapes you up, too. We all know that exercise trims the muscles, and that's very important in maintaining the slim look you want. But did you know that your soft, distended belly may in part be caused by poor circulation? That's right! If circulation is poor, blood can collect in the abdominal organs, causing them to bloat. Proper circulation keeps blood from congregating at any one point. So the first step in getting rid of your pot belly may be to get your heart in shape!

There's also a little-known benefit you can get from regular exercise that scientists are just beginning to learn about. When you engage in strenuous activity for a prolonged period of time, your brain produces tiny amounts of a chemical called *endorphin*. Endorphin is chemically similar to morphine, and it has a similar function—to help deaden pain and create a sense of euphoria. This explains the "high" long distance runners experience after many miles. It is the body's way of coping with the arduous task you've set for it. Researchers are discovering that regular exercise is the safest way of getting high.

Exercise can do hundreds of things for you, from preventing excess serum cholesterol, to curing impotence and frigidity, to clearing up acne. But you'll find out enough about these on your own. Let's turn now to a second important question: *How* should you exercise?

Study after study has shown that the most

effective types of exercise for weight loss are the
continuous nonstop rhythmical activities, such
as running, swimming, skating, skiing, hiking
and cycling[1] Your body must work strenuously
for a prolonged period in order to reach what is
called a negative caloric state; that is the point at
which your body begins to burn fat cells for
energy. "Spurty" activities, such as baseball, or
infrequent "weekend" sports such as golf have
been shown to be ineffective in bringing about
fat consumption. Only those activities which
keep you working will tone up your heart and
lungs and burn off fat.

Also, it's important that your exercise program
feature a variety of different exercises. The first
reason for this is physiological: each activity
builds a different set of muscles, and you need to
exercise *all* your muscles for good health.
Swimming strengthens different muscles than
jogging, cycling builds different muscles than
rowing. You ought to enjoy a variety of activities
in order to improve every muscle, blood vessel
and nerve in your body.

The second benefit of variety is psychological:
a varied exercise program is exciting. So many
people I talk to get bored with exercise and quit,
and I can understand why. They jog the same
block day in and day out. That sort of routine
isn't fun, it's a chore. And who needs another
chore? So when it comes to exercise, mix it up! It's
better for you   and a lot more enjoyable.

One of the best exercise routines we've found is
Jazzercise. It exercises and stretches every

muscle in the body in just 45 minutes. It is lots of fun, and will give you "energy." All aerobic programs are good, but Jazzercise seems to be the most fun.

The third thing to remember about exercise, especially at the beginning is to start slow, and day by day build your endurance. Your body needs time to firm up old muscle tissue and build new muscle and open up clogged arteries. If you try to do to much too soon, you can damage your joints, tendons and muscles. Even if you don't seriously damage yourself, the agony you'll experience will discourage you from keeping up with your exercise program. Easy does it! You'll have plenty of time to build up to a daily routine of moderately strenuous exercise. . .and you'll have a long, healthy life in which to enjoy all the super energy you'll get!

* * *

By now you've guessed that what I've proposed in this book is not really new diet plan. It is actually a new lifestyle! And this is as it should be; obesity, after all, is a way of life. Slimness and dynamic health, too, must be a way of life. After all, the very word "diet" comes from the greek word "diaita," meaning a way of living! [2]

But I hope I've convinced you that this new way of life is easier, cheaper and more exciting than the way you're living now. You'll enjoy every day more, you'll be more fully alive and turned on to the world around you. And best of all, you'll turn other people on too!

It really doesn't take much to sum up the recommendations I've made in this book. Forget calories. Instead, give your body what it's really asking for. Eat fresh, whole natural foods, which are high in nutritional density and life-giving fiber. Learn to tune in to your own body wisdom to meet your own nutritional needs. And finally, stay active.

I know this little prescription isn't as complex or technical as the ones you're used to hearing from the big-name diet doctors. But it's a plan that works. It's a plan you can live with.

And when I say live, I mean LIVE!

NOTES

[1] Thomas Kirk Cureton, *The Physiological Effects of Exercise Programs On Adults* (Springfield, Illinois: Charles C Thomas, 1969), p 52.

[2] Oscar E. Nybakken, *Greek and Latin In Scientific Terminology* (Ames, Iowa: Iowa State College Press, 1959), p. 160.

9

THOSE CRAZY DIETS
What's Wrong with the Diet You're Already On!

It seems that every time I tell people about the dangers and pitfalls of most weight loss diets, they are certain I'm not talking about THEIR diet. They're sure their own special program is the one that'll help them lose tens of pounds a week. So in this chapter, I'll name some names. I'll discuss some specific diets, and show you why they're ineffective, silly or even dangerous. As you read through the discussions, you'll notice that certain misconceptions keep cropping up again and again—the same myths I've already punctured!

*THE DOCTOR'S QUICK WEIGHT LOSS DIET (also known as the Stillman Diet or the Water Diet). Here's a meal plan which takes the high-protein concept to spectacularly absurd lengths. As I pointed out in the chapter on whole grains, the high-protein scam is based on the idea that since the body prefers burning carbohydrates to protein, the way to get rid of excess fat is to eat a lot of protein and not much carbohydrate. Your body is then supposed to go into "ketosis," wherein it burns body fat at a rapid rate.

In Stillman's diet, you eat no carbohydrates *at all*. You can eat as much as you like when it comes to lean meats, fish, chicken and turkey, seafoods, eggs and cottage cheese, but absolutely no carbohydrates.

There are two really big problems with this diet. In the first place, it presents a danger inherent in all low-carbohydrate diets: it robs the body of its best source of glucose, and thus stresses the liver, which must make glucose out of protein in order to keep the brain alive. And many experts feel that the ketosis this program is supposed to bring is not more effective that a more sensible weight-loss program.

Secondly, since the only allowed foods on the Stillman diet are from animal sources, the diet contains *no* fiber. Anyone who follows the diet for a significant period of time is setting him- or herself up for constipation, hemorrhoids, diverticulosis, etc. And *nobody* has suggested that the Stillman diet be followed for a lifetime.

*THE SCARSDALE DIET. Another high-protein plan, although this one does allow some carbohydrates and fiber. But the diet calls for too much meat (Monday's dinner calls for plenty of steak), this diet has an added booby-trap: black coffee, tea or diet soda is consumed at every meal. Caffeine is simply poison for those trying to curb their appetites.

* DR. ATKINS' DIET REVOLUTION. How a former heart specialist could have come up with this one is beyond me. It's the high-protein, low-

carbohydrate routine again, high in saturated fat and cholesterol, which are known contributors to atherosclerosis. There's a special gimmick with the Atkins plan—you test your urine constantly for the presence of ketones, and the idea is to keep the urine test stick the proper shade of purple (all this messing about in the potty may do more than anything else to help curb your appetite). According to Diet Digest, "If you still choose to follow this diet, we advise you to have a thorough physical examination and laboratory testing before the beginning."[1] I'd suggest you have your head examined while you're at it.

* THE SAVE YOUR LIFE DIET. This one is generally very excellent. Dr. David Reuben argues that the primary cause of obesity is lack of dietary fiber, and he has the evidence to back him up (certainly far more evidence than the ketone crowd has produced). I do have a few quibbles with him, however. In the first place, he seems to reject a whole-foods diet as the best way to insure proper fiber consumption. He writes disparagingly of trying to "regulate our diets by selecting only those foods with the highest roughage content from the grocer's shelves. That's a difficult assignment. . .Ninety-nine percent of American families will reject that regimen since they have been conditioned to the 'fashionable' and seductive low-roughage routine."[2]   Instead, Reuben suggests fortifying our processed food diet with a few spoonsful of

bran.

This is nonsense. It's easy to pick high-fiber foods; just stick with whole, natural foods, eat plenty of whole grain products, and avoid the stuff in the cans and boxes. A child could do it. "Ninety-nine percent of American families" would have only one conceivable excuse for rejecting such a regimen: sheer laziness.

Secondly, bran is not a fiber panacea. In the first place, bran does not contain the full range of dietary fibers. It's a very important fiber source, but it is completely lacking in soluble fibers, which are also crucial. Also, some studies indicate that isolated bran is not as effective as bran that's eaten as part of a whole-grain food. There is just no quick fix for our dietary fiber problems.

One more gripe: The Reuben diet allows coffee or tea at every meal. For shame!

*THE WOMAN DOCTOR'S DIET FOR WOMEN. An attempt to cash in on the women's movement. Dr. Barbara Edelstein argues that women tend to fail on most diets because most diets are designed by men. She apparently ignores the fact that those diets don't work for men, either. Otherwise, the "special women's diet" is quite conventional. There are some odd quirks, however: for instance, Dr. Edelstein allows you to substitute alcohol for a serving of fruit, the rawest nutritional deal I've ever heard of.

*THE CAMBRIDGE DIET. This latest low-calorie diet craze is causing controversy—and medical emergencies—all over the nation.

It's called the Cambridge Diet, named so because its inventor, Dr. Alan Howard, was a professor at Cambridge University, England. (Interestingly enough, Cambridge scientists have repudiated the diet, telling those who want to lose weight that they ought to eat whole, high-fiber foods instead!)[3] The diet purports to provide complete nutrition in only 330 calories a day. But doctors fear that it and other similar low-calorie diets may cause possibly fatal heart problems and other symptoms.

Specifically, the Cambridge Diet centers around a powdered mixture, a daily dose of which provides 33 grams of protein, 44 grams of carbohydrates (including fiber) and three grams of fat. The daily dose is also said to contain "100 percent of the USRDA for nutrients which for which a standard has been set."

An individual going on the diet is supposed to consume nothing but the diet for four weeks. After that, the dieter adds pre-planned meals of varying caloric content until the "optimum" caloric intake is determined.

On paper, it sounds marvelous. And indeed, the marketers of the Cambridge Diet claim that up to 20 pounds can be dropped in the first week. There's one problem, however—some people end up in the hospital before they can finish the diet.

The Food and Drug Administration has been keeping an eye on the fate of the Cambridge dieters, and is alarmed. FDA spokesman Jim Greene said that "The Cambridge Diet is not a diet a person should go on unless he or she is under medical supervision. We have documented cases of hospitalized people who were on the diet from three to six weeks. They suffered from dehydration, low blood pressure and cardiac irregularities." [4]

In an attempt to protect consumers from the hazards of the Cambridge Diet, the government has taken steps to control its marketing. In early 1980 the U.S. Postal Service charged that the distributors of the Cambridge Diet (The same folks who once brought you bust developers and other similar gew-gaws) had used the mails to exaggerate weight loss claims, and failed to warn of potential health risks. The U.S. District Court of Appeals in San Fransico issued a restraining order, and the distributors agreed to remove the objectionable statements and include a warning in their advertisements.

This warning statement, which appears on cans of Cambridge Diet formula, is forbidding. It reads: "Consult your doctor before starting this diet. In particular, individuals who have heart and cardiovascular conditions, stroke, kidney disease, diabetes, gout, hypoglycemia, chronic infections, the very elderly, growing children, adolescents, or anyone under medical care for any other condition should diet only under direct medical supervision. . .Pregnant women and nursing mothers should not be under any weight loss program."

The incredibly detailed warning should get the Cambridge Diet distributors off the hook legally— but is it of any practical value. After all, there are said to be more than half a million people on the Cambridge Diet in the U.S. alone—have all of them checked things out with their doctors? Are they under medical supervision now? The chances seems slim.

Personally, I have a lot of problems with the Cambridge Diet. The body simply isn't meant to lose up to a pound a day. And this business about providing the USRDA of vitamins and minerals that have had standards set for them is especially troubling. I've already talked about how bankrupt the USRDA is, in light of what we know about biochemical individuality. To say that the diet gives you 100 percent of the USRDA only says that chances are good you won't die of scurvy, beri-beri, pellagra or some other deficiency disease while you're on the diet. Big deal. There's no guarantee you'll get the nutrition YOU need for good health—in fact, it would be pretty surprising if you did. People do lose weight on the Cambridge plan, but it's unsafe to stay on it.

*WEIGHT LOSS GIMMICKS. There are so many of these I'd need more than a book to cover them all—I'd need an encyclopedia. Let me knock down a few of the major ones, anyway.

One of the oldest tricks in the book is the PASSIVE WEIGHT LOSS DEVICE. The idea here is that you can trim down without exercising and without dieting—all you have to do is wrap, strap or clap yourself into the device. There's lots of different kinds: the old vibrating belt, weight loss creams, plastic girdles or suits, body-wrapping and hundreds of others. They've been going in and out of style, but you're guaranteed to find ads for at least one in the back pages of any women's magazine.

There's one thing you can say for sure about genuine passive weight loss devices—there aren't any. The only way to get rid of fat is to aerobically expend more energy than you take in, so that the body is forced to call upon its energy stores. There's nothing passive about the way you put on all that weight—haw can there possibly be a way to take it off passively?

But don't the venders of these toys have testimonials, even eye-witness demonstrations, to prove they work? Frequently they do, but these success stories can be attributed to three causes:

Water loss. Many of the passive devices—like plastic pants and saunas—make you sweat. All the water you lose weighs something, and so the bathroom scale may show you're a few pounds lighter. But don't think you've lost any fat; you almost certainly haven't, and the water weight will come back again in a few hours.

Diet and Exercise. Many of the gimmicks are accompanied by a "special diet and exercise program," and any weight lost is almost certainly due to sticking to the program, device or no device.

Lies. Very few of the success claims made by passive device peddlers have every been verified, and many of those that have have been found fraudulent. There are lots of things you shouldn't swallow when you're trying to slim down—and advertising hype is one of them.

Another popular weight-loss gimmick is the DIET PILL. These pill come in two types: the kind that are supposed to curb your appetite so you stay on your diet, and some newer varieties which are supposed to let you eat whatever you want and still lose weight.

Appetite-curbing pills are available by prescription (mostly amphetamines) or over-the-counter (stimulants). Amphetamines work by generally stimulating the central nervous system. While it's thought that amphetamines help weight loss by inhibiting appetite, there's no evidence that that's precisely how they help. Amphetamine diet pills can cause abnormal heart rates, high blood pressure, restlessness, dizziness, insomnia, euphoria, tremor, headache, psychotic episodes, dryness of mouth, diarrhea, constipation, allergic reactions, impotence, loss of sex drive—and, most important, they are extremely addictive.[5] Medical sources like the PHYSICIAN'S DESK REFERENCE recommend that amphetamines only be used as a last resort—and certainly no one who had not tried a whole-foods diet has any excuse for taking them.

Stimulants are a bit safer, but not much. In fact, there's some agreement that if one of the most common diet-aid stimulants, caffeine, had been discovered recently rather than thousands of years ago, it would be available only by prescription. [6] Stimulants work by causing the adrenals to excrete insulin, which in turn makes the body convert glycogen into glucose. So stimulants actually work to raise blood sugar levels, thus helping to stave off hunger and provide the lift so many dieters need.

Sounds great, right? Actually, there are a lot of problems involved in this kind of appetite control. In the first place, if they are used in conjunction with a processed food diet, these diet pills only serve to help you eat *less processed food,* so you provide your body with even less of what it needs to feel healthy and satisfied. This only worsens hunger. Also, that artificially-raised blood sugar level will drop eventually; then what happens? Your body signals the brain that blood sugar levels must be lifted again, and the result is hunger. That's why even though stimulants like caffeine are appetite suppressants in the short run, in the long run they are some of the most effective appetite *stimulants* known. So what we said about caffeine-laden diet sodas in an earlier chapter goes doubly true for caffeine-laced diet pills: pass 'em by.

Another popular over-the counter appetite suppressant—phenylpropanolamine hydrochloride—has problems of its own. It is recommended that individuals with high blood pressure, heart disease, diabetes or thyroid disease, or who are taking prescription drugs, not take phenylpropanolamine unless under a doctor's direction. Once again, it is unlikely that many of millions of people who take these preparations (such as Dexatrim, Obestat and Prolamine) ever seek such medical advice. Yet if they are overweight, the chances are very good that they do suffer from at least one of these ailments. Further, if the recommended dosage of phenylpropanolamine is exceeded, you may suffer rapid pulse, high blood pressure, nervousness, restlessness or sleeplessness.[7] I'd take being a little paunchy any day.

There's a new gimmick diet pill on the market (at least it's still on the market as we go to press, despite the fact that it was banned by the FDA in July, 1982), called Starch Blockers. Starch Blockers are composed of an enzyme derived from beans which is said to prevent the absorption of complex carbohydrates in the intestine, so you don't get calories from them. In a way, then, the starch blockers are just a new version of the low-carbohydrate diet. But instead of restricting you to protein, the pill restricts the availability of carbohydrate, so that you can eat your cake and still not "have" it.

The jury is still out on starch blockers—way, way out. The FDA hasn't even tested them for safety yet, much less for effectiveness. There are plenty of unanswered questions concerning starch blockers. For instance, if a low- or no-carbohydrate diet is unsafe (and we have seen that it is), is it safe to radically restrict the absorption of carbohydrates? What other side-effects can this tampering with carbohydrate metabolism create? Some doctors I know are convinced that starch blocker users are more prone to kidney stones, and the FDA has received complaints that the pills cause nausea and other unpleasant symptoms. Although starch blockers block complex carbohydrates, they do not limit the absorption of simple carbohydrates, which are much more dangerous to the dieter.

And there's one question which particularly bothers me: what's supposed to *happen* to all that unabsorbed carbohydrate? Just look at all the foods you're supposed to be able to eat when you take starch blockers: soft white bread, pasta, sweet rolls, cake...All of these are *low fiber* foods. Apparently, then, taking starch blockers greatly increases the amount of low-fiber undigested material in the intestine. What's to keep all this low-fiber digesta from compacting in the colon, increasing the danger of constipation, diverticular disease and colon cancer? And how many millions of bottles of starch-blockers will be sold before we find out?

I have a more fundamental objection to starch blockers, and it is the same objection that I have with all of the get-thin-quick diets and pills and gimmicks. Losing weight is simply one facet of returning to your normal metabolic balance. As such, it ought to be a *natural* process, a process involving natural nourishment and natural activity, a process which follows the body's own rhythms. All of the diets and drugs and programs we looked at in this chapter are really efforts to *cheat,* to get the body to speed up its use of fat while we sit around gorging ourselves and not doing a lick of work. They are attempts to fool the body; but we need to remember that the body is seldom fooled. Its rules and rhythms must be kept, or disaster follows. Someone ought to tell the purveyors of the protein diets and the pill pushers and the starch blocker sellers that the human organism did not survive and dominate this planet for hundreds of thousands of years by being as dopey as they make it out to be!

NOTES

[1] *Diet Digest Rates The Diets,* Vol. 1 No. 2, 1981, p. 19.

[2] David Reuben, *The Save Your Life Diet* (New York: Ballantine Books, 1975), p. 81.

[3] Barbara Mullarkey, "The Cambridge Diet: Caution," *Vegetarian Times,* September 1982, pp. 32-33.

[4] Ibid.

[5] 1981 *Physician's Desk Reference* (Oradell, New Jersey)

10

YOUR BODY WISDOM DIARY

We introduced the concept of body wisdom in Chapter Four. Body wisdom means becoming aware of all the signals by which you body tells you how it's doing. Tens of thousands of years before the age of doctors, these physical messages helped us stay alive in the face of a hostile environment. And even today, a physicians first tool in making a diagnosis is (or ought to be) the question, "How do you feel?" Your Body Wisdom Diary will tell you the same thing for a lot less money.

Lost in the fairyland of commercial media and deluged with easy-to-get, over-the-counter drugs, we face the ultimate alienation: we have lost touch with our own bodies. We feel a headache, indigestion, constipation or any number of aches and pains, but we do not ask ourselves, "What's wrong? What have I done to make my body complain? What must I do to feel well again?" Instead, we reach for aspirin, antacids, laxatives and other potent chemicals in order to attain, not a state of health, but a drugged numbness which we have been taught to equate with "feeling better."

It is time to get in touch with ourselves once again. In a sense, it is simply not enough to say "listen to what your body tells you." We have been wandering in an alien limbo, halfway between sickness and health, for so long that we no longer recognize our native language. We must re-learn body wisdom. To help you experience your body's message, I have developed this 14-day Body Wisdom Diary. It will help you keep track of your body's reactions to the food you eat for two weeks. Although the process, if followed faithfully, is rather pain-staking, it will reveal valuable insights into your unique metabolism. I'll bet your body has some pretty surprising things to say!

There are two steps involved in filling out the Body Wisdom Diary. You'll notice that each page of the diary is marked out in hours (a.m. on the left-hand pages, p.m. on the right) and that each page is divided down the middle. On the left half, you are to record *what you eat.* And here I mean everything your eat—your main meals as well as your little snacks throughout the day. Include also what you drink, and any drugs— prescription or over-the-counter—that you may take. Be as specific as you can. Mention brand names when possible; not all apple juices, for example, are created equal, and some brands may cause negative reactions while others do not.

Simply filling out this half of the diary will be an education in itself. It may be the first time you've ever seen your dietary lifestyle laid out in front of you! As the nutritional picture develops, pay attention to certain features:

*Is your diet high in refined carbohydrates (white sugar, white flour)?

*Do you tend to eat the same few foods time and time again?

*Do you eat a lot of processed foods?

*Is your diet heavy in chemical additives?

*Is your breakfast scanty?

*Is your supper heavy?

*Are your snacks "junkier" than your meals?

*When are you most likely to snack?

*When are you most likely to drink alcohol?

*When are you most likely to binge? Make a note of these, and note also any other abnormalities in your dietary pattern.

The second step in completing the Body Wisdom Diary is to note *how you feel.* This step is especially important if you are using the Body Wisdom Diary in connection with the Rotation Diet and food testing which we described in Chapter 6. Once again, the more specific you are, the more useful the Body Wisdom Diary becomes. Make a note of any physical or emotional ups and downs during the day, and be sure to record the hour at which you first noticed them. Take special notice of the following negative signs:

1) Mental confusion

2) Difficulty in concentration

3) Temper tantrums or other uncontrolled emotions

4) Sexual impotence or frigidity

5) Depression

6) Nervousness

7) Blurred or double vision

8) Dizziness or fainting spells

9) Exhaustion

10) Sleepiness or inability to sleep

11) Extreme tiredness upon arising

12) Cold sweats

13) Craving for alcohol, coffee, cigarettes or other drugs

14) Constipation or diarrhea

15) Abdominal distress

16) Loss of appetite or extreme hunger

17) Headaches

18) Flare-up of any skin problems

19) Excessive perspiration

20) Outbreaks of allergies or asthma

21) Catching a cold

22) Aching joints

23) Cramps

24) Cravings for specific foods (be sure to note what kind of food you craved) For convenience, you may simply write the number of the symptom in the provided blank. You'll also need to make a note of your body's positive signals:

25) A feeling of happiness and well-being

26) Waking up feeling refreshed in the morning

27) Being satisfied with a moderate amount of food

28) Physical strength

29) Disappearance of a physical ailment

30) Calmness

31) Sexual ability and enjoyment

32) Mental alertness In other words, mark down those times when you say to yourself, "Hey, I really feel great!"

When you have completed two weeks of observations, study your diary carefully. Do any patterns emerge? For instance:

*When your meals are high in refined carbohydrates and other processed foods, do you feel hunger or the need for a stimulant at mid-morning and mid-afternoon? Which foods tend to satisfy these feelings, and which do not?

*Is an evening of junk-food snacking followed by weakness or tiredness in the morning?

*Do you feel headachy, nervous or hyperactive after eating foods high in chemical additives or refined carbohydrates?

*Do some foods cause flare-ups of physical ailments, such as acne? Do some foods tend to give relief for these problems?

*After what kinds of meals are you most likely to feel healthy and energetic?

Now, I'm not saying these patterns will develop for you, or even that they should. Your metabolism is unique, so your nutritional responses will be one-of-a-kind as well. The Body Wisdom Diary is simply meant to help you become aware of your body's responses .

And now that you ARE aware of you body's reaction to foods, just eat those things that make you feel good, and avoid those things that make you feel good, and avoid those things that make you feel bad. What could be more healthful?

BODY WISDOM DIARY

WEEK ONE	A.M.	DAY ONE
TIME	WHAT I ATE	HOW I FELT
1:00		
2:00		
3:00		
4:00		
5:00		
6:00		
7:00		
8:00		
9:00		
10:00		
11:00		
12:00		

BODY WISDOM DIARY

WEEK ONE	P.M.	DAY ONE
TIME	WHAT I ATE	HOW I FELT

TIME	WHAT I ATE	HOW I FELT
1:00		
2:00		
3:00		
4:00		
5:00		
6:00		
7:00		
8:00		
9:00		
10:00		
11:00		
12:00		

BODY WISDOM DIARY

WEEK ONE	A.M.	DAY TWO
TIME	WHAT I ATE	HOW I FELT
1:00		
2:00		
3:00		
4:00		
5:00		
6:00		
7:00		
8:00		
9:00		
10:00		
11:00		
12:00		

BODY WISDOM DIARY

WEEK ONE	P.M.	DAY TWO

TIME	WHAT I ATE	HOW I FELT
1:00		
2:00		
3:00		
4:00		
5:00		
6:00		
7:00		
8:00		
9:00		
10:00		
11:00		
12:00		

BODY WISDOM DIARY

WEEK ONE	A.M.	DAY THREE
TIME	WHAT I ATE	HOW I FELT
1:00		
2:00		
3:00		
4:00		
5:00		
6:00		
7:00		
8:00		
9:00		
10:00		
11:00		
12:00		

BODY WISDOM DIARY

WEEK ONE	P.M.	DAY THREE
TIME	WHAT I ATE	HOW I FELT

TIME	WHAT I ATE	HOW I FELT
1:00		
2:00		
3:00		
4:00		
5:00		
6:00		
7:00		
8:00		
9:00		
10:00		
11:00		
12:00		

BODY WISDOM DIARY

WEEK ONE	A.M.	DAY FOUR
TIME	WHAT I ATE	HOW I FELT
1:00		
2:00		
3:00		
4:00		
5:00		
6:00		
7:00		
8:00		
9:00		
10:00		
11:00		
12:00		

BODY WISDOM DIARY

WEEK ONE	P.M.	DAY FOUR

TIME	WHAT I ATE	HOW I FELT
1:00		
2:00		
3:00		
4:00		
5:00		
6:00		
7:00		
8:00		
9:00		
10:00		
11:00		
12:00		

BODY WISDOM DIARY

WEEK ONE	A.M.	DAY FIVE
TIME	WHAT I ATE	HOW I FELT
1:00		
2:00		
3:00		
4:00		
5:00		
6:00		
7:00		
8:00		
9:00		
10:00		
11:00		
12:00		

BODY WISDOM DIARY

WEEK ONE	P.M.	DAY FIVE
TIME	WHAT I ATE	HOW I FELT

TIME	WHAT I ATE	HOW I FELT
1:00		
2:00		
3:00		
4:00		
5:00		
6:00		
7:00		
8:00		
9:00		
10:00		
11:00		
12:00		

BODY WISDOM DIARY

<u>WEEK ONE</u>   A.M.   <u>DAY SIX</u>

TIME	WHAT I ATE	HOW I FELT
1:00		
2:00		
3:00		
4:00		
5:00		
6:00		
7:00		
8:00		
9:00		
10:00		
11:00		
12:00		

BODY WISDOM DIARY

WEEK ONE   P.M.   DAY SIX

TIME	WHAT I ATE	HOW I FELT
1:00		
2:00		
3:00		
4:00		
5:00		
6:00		
7:00		
8:00		
9:00		
10:00		
11:00		
12:00		

BODY WISDOM DIARY

WEEK ONE	A.M.	DAY SEVEN
TIME	WHAT I ATE	HOW I FELT
1:00		
2:00		
3:00		
4:00		
5:00		
6:00		
7:00		
8:00		
9:00		
10:00		
11:00		
12:00		

BODY WISDOM DIARY

WEEK ONE	P.M.	DAY SEVEN
TIME	WHAT I ATE	HOW I FELT
1:00		
2:00		
3:00		
4:00		
5:00		
6:00		
7:00		
8:00		
9:00		
10:00		
11:00		
12:00		

BODY WISDOM DIARY

WEEK TWO	A.M.	DAY ONE
TIME	WHAT I ATE	HOW I FELT
1:00		
2:00		
3:00		
4:00		
5:00		
6:00		
7:00		
8:00		
9:00		
10:00		
11:00		
12:00		

BODY WISDOM DIARY

WEEK TWO	P.M.	DAY ONE

TIME	WHAT I ATE	HOW I FELT
1:00		
2:00		
3:00		
4:00		
5:00		
6:00		
7:00		
8:00		
9:00		
10:00		
11:00		
12:00		

BODY WISDOM DIARY

WEEK TWO	A.M.	DAY TWO
TIME	WHAT I ATE	HOW I FELT
1:00		
2:00		
3:00		
4:00		
5:00		
6:00		
7:00		
8:00		
9:00		
10:00		
11:00		
12:00		

BODY WISDOM DIARY

WEEK TWO	P.M.	DAY TWO

TIME	WHAT I ATE	HOW I FELT
1:00		
2:00		
3:00		
4:00		
5:00		
6:00		
7:00		
8:00		
9:00		
10:00		
11:00		
12:00		

BODY WISDOM DIARY

WEEK TWO	A.M.	DAY THREE
TIME	WHAT I ATE	HOW I FELT
1:00		
2:00		
3:00		
4:00		
5:00		
6:00		
7:00		
8:00		
9:00		
10:00		
11:00		
12:00		

BODY WISDOM DIARY

WEEK TWO	P.M.	DAY THREE
TIME	WHAT I ATE	HOW I FELT
1:00		
2:00		
3:00		
4:00		
5:00		
6:00		
7:00		
8:00		
9:00		
10:00		
11:00		
12:00		

BODY WISDOM DIARY

WEEK TWO	A.M.	DAY FOUR
TIME	WHAT I ATE	HOW I FELT

TIME	WHAT I ATE	HOW I FELT
1:00		
2:00		
3:00		
4:00		
5:00		
6:00		
7:00		
8:00		
9:00		
10:00		
11:00		
12:00		

BODY WISDOM DIARY

WEEK TWO	P.M.	DAY FOUR
TIME	WHAT I ATE	HOW I FELT
1:00		
2:00		
3:00		
4:00		
5:00		
6:00		
7:00		
8:00		
9:00		
10:00		
11:00		
12:00		

BODY WISDOM DIARY

WEEK TWO	A.M.	DAY FIVE
TIME	WHAT I ATE	HOW I FELT
1:00		
2:00		
3:00		
4:00		
5:00		
6:00		
7:00		
8:00		
9:00		
10:00		
11:00		
12:00		

BODY WISDOM DIARY

WEEK TWO	P.M.	DAY FIVE
TIME	WHAT I ATE	HOW I FELT
1:00		
2:00		
3:00		
4:00		
5:00		
6:00		
7:00		
8:00		
9:00		
10:00		
11:00		
12:00		

BODY WISDOM DIARY

WEEK TWO	A.M.	DAY SIX
TIME	WHAT I ATE	HOW I FELT
1:00		
2:00		
3:00		
4:00		
5:00		
6:00		
7:00		
8:00		
9:00		
10:00		
11:00		
12:00		

BODY WISDOM DIARY

WEEK TWO	P.M.	DAY SIX

TIME	WHAT I ATE	HOW I FELT
1:00		
2:00		
3:00		
4:00		
5:00		
6:00		
7:00		
8:00		
9:00		
10:00		
11:00		
12:00		

BODY WISDOM DIARY

WEEK TWO	A.M.	DAY SEVEN
TIME	WHAT I ATE	HOW I FELT
1:00		
2:00		
3:00		
4:00		
5:00		
6:00		
7:00		
8:00		
9:00		
10:00		
11:00		
12:00		

BODY WISDOM DIARY

WEEK TWO	P.M.	DAY SEVEN
TIME	WHAT I ATE	HOW I FELT
1:00		
2:00		
3:00		
4:00		
5:00		
6:00		
7:00		
8:00		
9:00		
10:00		
11:00		
12:00		

11

FRINGE BENEFITS

A diet that helps you lose weight, meets all your nutritional needs, fights off hunger, saves you money, and frees you from counting calories or carbohydrates. . .this alone is the answer to the dreams of millions of overweight people across the country. I promise the simple program I've laid out here will help you do all these things.

But there's a lot more that a whole foods diet can do for you. Remember, your body was made to thrive on whole grains and fresh fruits and vegetables, so it's no surprise that a diet of natural foods is good for your whole body. . .not just your waistline. Following the nutritional principles I've set down here will not only make you thinner, but it will bring new life to your entire system!

Here are just some of the extra benefits a whole goods diet will bring you: BETTER SEX

I bet THAT makes your eyes light up! And why not? Sex has always been very important to humans as individuals and as a species. Sexuality is a fundamental part of our very consciousness. People are right to be concerned about it.

But it seems more people are worried about sex than ever before. And statistics indicate these problems are real. Recent studies show male sperm counts have been dropping steadily over the last 20 years.[1] A 1978 survey of 100 volunteer couples suggests that sexual problems are now quite frequent, even among the happily married. Of the women studied, 15 percent reported inability to have an orgasm, while fully 46 percent described some difficulty in reaching orgasm.

Among the men, 16 percent reported difficulty in attaining or maintaining an erection, and 36 percent reported premature ejaculation. Thirty-five percent of the women and 12 percent of the men said they were disinterested in sex, and 28 percent of women and 10 percent of the men said they were "turned off" sexually.[2] A growing number of people simply aren't happy with their sex lives.

A great handicap here is the tendency of most people to thing of sexual problems as emotional problems rather than as physical ailments. Certainly psychology has its place, but it must be remembered that sex is fundamentally a physical and physiological process. Good sex is impossible without good health.

And, as I've already pointed out, good health is impossible without good nutrition. The link between sex and nutrition is well-recognized. One of this country's leading neuropharmacologists, Dr. Carl C. Pfeiffer, director of the

Brain Bio Center in New Jersey, reports that vitamin deficiencies are "the most common cause of impotency in the young male and amenorrhea (lack of menstruation) in the female."[3] Most important in this regard are Zinc, which plays a vital role in sperm and ova production, and vitamin B6. Writes Pfeiffer, "Certainly, patients both male and female whom we have seen for problems of lack of menses, potency and fertility have successfully produced children when their zinc and vitamin B6 deficiency was corrected."[4]

Also connected with proper sexual function is the substance histamine, which plays a role in male ejaculation and orgasm in both sexes. Histamine levels are related to the presence of the nutrient folic acid. Pfeiffer has noted that the use of folic acid to elevate blood and tissue histamine will provide easier orgasm in the low-histamine female[5]

Of all the nutrients vital to sexual function, vitamin E has perhaps received the most attention. Although the evidence for humans is less clear, early research indicates that vitamin E plays an important role in reproduction[6]

Zinc, folic acid, vitamins B6 and E. All these, and many others, are needed for good sex. Yet it is precisely these that are stolen from processed foods. Any heat at all tends to destroy B6, and vitamin E is discarded with the natural oils that are removed from foods to extend shelf life. Take a look at the figures for white bread, for instance. "Enriched" white bread contains less than half the zinc found in whole wheat bread. It also contains just one-fifth the B6, and 37 percent less folic acid.[7] The wheat germ, rich in vitamin E, is also removed from white flour.

Given all this, it's a little hard to understand why Americans are willing to waste millions of dollars on zany therapies and semipornagraphic manuals and at the same time stuff garbage into their mouths which almost guarantees sexual frustration. Looking at sexy pictures won't put zinc and B6 into your food. Only a whole foods diet can proved the nutrition you need for a happy sex life.

BEAT HEART DISEASE

I was a bit surprised as I turned from my study of diet and sex to review the literature on diet and heart disease. It seemed that all you had to do was replace the word "impotency" with "arteriosclerosis," and it was like reading the same material all over again! No wonder there's a link between heart disease and impotency![8]

Vitamin E, B6 and folic acid are implicated here once again. Vitamin B6 helps the body keep its serum cholesterol levels low, and it is of course high serum cholesterol which is responsible for fatty deposits in coronary arteries which leads to heart attack. Monkeys on a B6-deficient diet rapidly develop atherosclerosis, and the same thing seems to be true for other members of the animal kingdom. The role of vitamin E in the prevention and cure of heart disease, and folic acid, a substance which promotes histamine production and thus better circulation, has been shown to diminish atherosclerotic conditions in the elderly?[9]

Other nutrients also help fight heart disease. Lecithin is an effective emulsifying agent—that is, it keeps cholesterol deposits from forming and helps remove those that have formed. The body produces its own lecithin, although supplements are available. Proper consumption of choline—present in whole foods—helps the body keep its lecithin levels up.[10] Vitamin C helps build collagen, a protein which is indispensable to heart tissues and blood vessels. Prison camp victims with vitamin C deficiencies have been found to suffer from wide-spread fatty deposits in their arteries.[11]

As a matter of fact, since bodily functions involve whole complexes of nutrients working together, a deficiency in ANY nutrient can contribute to heart disease. I can only repeat that the best way to develop a nutrient deficiency is to eat processed foods. The best way to avoid nutrient deficiencies—and heart disease—is to eat a whole, natural foods diet.

No one talks about it much, but the nutrient that may be the most effective in preventing heart disease is the secret nutrient: *fiber*.

I mentioned earlier that fiber tends to increase fat excretion. Fiber has also been shown to cut serum cholesterol levels dramatically. In one recent study, patients on a high-fiber diet lowered there cholesterol levels by 35 percent, and their triglyceride levels by 65 percent![12]

One more point. The Working Group on

Arteriosclerosis of the National Heart, Lung and Blood institute has recommended that you cut down on your consumption of fats, especially saturated fats, to decrease the risk of heart disease.[13] I have but one addition to this very sound advice. Processed foods are generally high in saturated fats. The food scientists know that fat is a cheap ingredient, it adds weight to foods, and it stimulates the appetite, so they add it to foods whenever and wherever they can get away with it. Whole grains and fresh fruits and vegetables are very low in fat. Enough said!

AVOID CANCER

Interestingly enough, the absence of both halves of our hunger equation— nutritional density and fiber—have been implicated in cancer.

We've already talked a bit about fiber and cancer, but let's say a little more. Two groups of bacteria which regularly infest the average human's stomach are the bacterioids and bifidobacteria. These bacteria can convert the bile acid cholic acid into the potent carcinogen apcholic acid, and another bile acid, deoxycholic acid, into one of the most powerful cancer-causing agent known, 3-methyl-cholanthrene. If low-fiber fecal material remains in contact with the intestinal wall for a prolonged period, malignancies are likely to develop.[14] Fecal matter high in fiber, however, moves swiftly through the intestine and prevents this cancer-causing contact. As we've said, whole foods are high-fiber foods.

Other nutrients have been linked to cancer prevention as well. Selenium, present in wheat germ, bran, onions, tomatoes and broccoli is thought to neutralize certain carcinogens and provide protection from some cancers. Once again, selenium's worst enemies are food processing techniques.[15] (A note about selenium: if you're on a whole foods diet, you're bound to get all the selenium you need. Use supplements only under a doctor's supervision, because selenium overdose can be toxic!)

Massachusetts Institute of Technology researchers have discovered that vitamins C and E, along with certain other whole-foods micronutrients called indoles, are also effective in inhibiting carcinogens.[16] And of course Nobel Laureate Dr. Linus Pauling is one of the world's leading proponents of vitamin C as a cancer-fighting nutrient.

All in all, hundreds of doctors have echoed the sentiments of Dr. J.R. Davidson, former associate professor of clinical medicine at the University of Manitoba, who wrote, "I believe cancer, a deficiency disease, can be prevented and controlled by a suitable and balanced diet, high in vitamin content."[17]

These are just three of the diseases you can avoid if you stick to a whole foods diet. There are more; natural foods can help you lick alcoholism, allergies, anemia, arthritis, asthma, backache, high blood pressure, constipation, fatigue, indigestion, infections, insomnia, leg cramps, ulcers. . .and on and on and on!

Right now you're probably saying, "Wait a minute! This fellow Stitt sounds like he's selling one of those quack medicines that are supposed to cure everything! Isn't he going a little overboard with this natural foods business?"

Let me answer you directly. Yes, I believe that whole foods will bring the benefits I've mentioned to almost every person, almost every time. But my optimism isn't based on quackery, but on common scientific sense. The human organism developed and reached it's present state eating whole, fresh, natural foods. Whole foods are what we're *built* to run on. Thus it stands to reason that a whole foods diet will keep us healthy.

Let me draw a little analogy. An automobile, of course, it built to run on gasoline. If you started to add water and sand to your gas, and if you lowered the octane level of the fuel so that it burned less efficiently, it wouldn't be long before every major part of your engine would be ruined. Yet no one finds it strange that you can avoid corrosion, cylinder wear, engine knock, dieseling, fuel line freeze up and abysmal gas mileage simply by using the right fuel! Why then do so many doubt that most illnesses can be avoided simply by eating the right food?

Have I convinced you? Have I broken down all your objections? I hope so. I hope I've shown you that all you thought you knew about diets is wrong. More importantly, I hope I convinced you that whole, natural foods are the answer to your diet problems.

So come on! Start to turn your diet around today. Follow the principles I've set down here, and be sure and let me know how they work for you. Because if there's one thing I hope you've learned in this book it is this: a whole-foods diet is not just the key to a brand new waistline; it's the door to a whole new life!

NOTES

[1] "Sperm Gap," *East-West Journal,* December 1981, p. 14.

[2] E. Frank, C. Anderson, D. Rubinstein, "Frequency of sexual dysfunction in 'normal' couples," *New England Journal of Medicine,* Vol. 299, 1978, pp. 111-115.

[3] Carl C. Pfeiffer, *Mental and Elemental Nutrients* (New Canaan, Connecticut: Keats Publishing Inc., 1975), p. 469.

[4] Pfeiffer, p. 471

[5] Pfeiffer, p. 472

[6] P.E. Norris, *About Wheat Germ* (Wellingborough, Northamptonshire, U.K.: Thorsons Publishers Limited, 1975), p. 29.

[7] Tom Gorman, "Now we know—wheat does beat white," *Bakery,* June 1981, p. 53.

[8] Robert C. Kolodny, William H. Masters, Virginia E. Johnson and Mae A. Biggs, *Textbook of Human Sexuality For Nurses* (Boston: Little, Brown and Company, 1979), p. 376.

[9] Roger J. Williams, *Nutrition Against Disease* (New York: Bantam Books, 1971), pp. 77-78.

[10] Williams, p. 76.

[11] Williams, p. 85.

[12] D. Kritchevsky, S.A. Tepper and J.A. Story, "Nonnutritive Fiber and Lipid Metabolism," *Journal of Food Science,* Vol. 40, 1975, pp. 8-11.

[13] Working Group on Arteriosclerosis of the National Heart, Lung and Blood Institute, *Arteriosclerosis* 1981, Vol. 1 (Washington D.C.: National Institute on Health Publication No. 81-2034, June 1981), p. 33.

[14] David Reuben, *The Save Your Life Diet* (New York: Ballantine Books, 1976), p. 30.

[15] Earl Mindell, *Earl Mindell's Vitamin Bible* (New York: Rawson, Wade Publishers Inc., 1979), p. 88.

[16] Mindell, p. 15.

[17] Linda Clark, *Get Well Naturally* (New York: Arco Publishing Company Inc., 1965), p. 226.

12

GETTING HIGH
Relieving the Stress that
Makes you Eat

There's a different kind of eating problem we haven't dealt with yet—the problem of stress-related eating. In a way, this kind of difficulty falls outside the normal realm of dieting because the solution to stress-induced eating lies not in satisfying your hunger, but developing more positive strategies to deal with stress.

And stress *can* make you eat. Studies with human subjects repeatedly show that emotional or physical stress can increase food consumption. In the past, this phenomenon was explained in terms of upbringing; food was given to children as a reward for being "good," so that they learn to associate food with emotional acceptance. As adults, then, we tent to eat when we feel the need for support and acceptance.

But recent research indicates that the tendency to respond to stress by eating may have a more rudimentary biochemical basis. Rats, when subjected to stress in the form of tail-pinching, will eat ravenously, even when not previously deprived of food. The reaction seems to involve several distinct mechanism; when satiety is induced through naxolone injections, the rats continue to chew, and may completely demolish food even though they won't swallow any.

In humans, of course, sources of stress are seldom so specific as a pinch on the tail. Kinesiolgists tell us that each of us has a stress threshold. Our bodies can cope with all sorts of disturbances without showing troublesome symptoms. But all these shocks are stored up, and eventually even the slightest stress can push us over our threshold. Then the brain send out what are called "dysponetic signals"—signs with tell the body to react to crisis.

These dysponetic signals, of course, served an important purpose for our primate ancestors. When faced with an onrushing lion, for instance, even the most laid-back Neanderthal would leap over his or her stress threshold. Then the body's fight-or-flee system would brace the muscles, pump adrenaline into the system, and increase blood flow to vital organs. Our shaggy forebear would then be able to take immediate and specific action.

But today we tend to creep over our stress thresholds, inching toward it shock by shock. The stress which sends us over may be nothing more serious than a flat tire or a thoughtless criticism from the boss—but our bodies are braced for desperate action. There's no specific action to take—you can hardly flee from a flat or punch your boss— so the tension stores up in your body.

All this stored tension can do more than just make you eat. Your continually disturbed and tensed muscles no longer return to their proper resting positions. If these muscles go into spasm, they may press on blood vessels and nerves, causing poor circulation and numbness or pain. Continuous stress can also lead to migraine-like headaches, muscle-contraction headaches, neckaches and backaches, poor circulation in hands, legs and feet and internal disorders like high blood pressure and ulcers.

What do we do to cope with stress? Increasingly, we exhibit a different kind of fleeing behavior: flight from the world itself. We turn to alcohol and other drugs to "turn off" our stressful lives. The number of adult regular alcohol users increased more than 12 percent in the five years preceding 1979. More than a third of these drank five or more drinks at a sitting. But for adults, marijuana is by far the fastest-growing high. Its use increased 200 percent during the same period.

Among young adults, perhaps the most stressed segment of our society, drug abuse is hardly less an epidemic than it was in the 1960s. During the 1974-1979 period, cocaine use among young adults increased 200 percent, and sedative use was up 75 percent. The number of regular marijuana users increased 40 percent, of hallucinogenic drugs, 20 percent, and of alcohol, 8 percent. As these young adults mature and take their places in the job market, they will no doubt be even more prone than their parents to turn to chemical relief from stress.

Obviously, the use of alcohol and other drugs is a very destructive means of stress management. Heavy and continual use of alcohol can lead to alcoholism, a pernicious and life-shortening addiction. But that's not all; alcohol abusers are also prone to high blood pressure, cancers of the esophagus, stomach, head and neck, increased susceptibility to infection, decreased sex drive, impotence and menstrual irregularity.

Marijuana, despite its reputation as a safe high, is no less damaging to those who turn to it regularly. Studies indicate that marijuana smoking increases the heart's work-load, decreases usable volume of the lungs, damages lung tissue (far more than does tobacco), decreases motivation and may contribute to sex hormone imbalance. And cocaine, a drug that's making a big come-back in the U.S., can contribute to disorders ranging from the deterioration of nasal tissue to psychotic episodes.

The fact that these traditional methods of escape are so dangerous does nothing to relieve our dilemma. We are all under incredible stress: stress that makes us sick, stress that may make us overeat. We've *got* to find relief. We've got to have a way to turn off our troubles and enter a more relaxed, serene state of consciousness. Once in a while, every one of us has got to get high.

Fortunately, there are natural, healthy ways

to get high—and they really work! These intoxicating strategies fall into two categories: exercise and deep relaxation.

Exercise works to get you high in two ways. In the first place, it improves you body's ability to cope with stress. Regular strenuous exercise helps release all that tension that's building up inside you. Plus, exercise slows the pulse, increases heart and lung efficiency, lowers the blood pressure and slow the basal metabolic rate.

Very importantly, exercise increases the the supply of the oxygen to the brain. As a brain researcher Peter Russel points out, "Oxygen is essential to brain function. Although the brain amounts to only two percent of the body's weight, it consumes 25 percent of the body's oxygen intake. If the oxygen supply is reduced, brain function suffers." It is precisely the increased cardio-pulmonary-vascular efficiency that exercise brings which helps improve the brain's oxygen supply. And a well-supplied brain feels good!

Just through the rather simple process of improving the body's vital functions, then, exercise provides a good escape from stress. Russel confirms, "Exercise can also directly affect personality. Regular jogging and physical training lead not only to physical fitness but also to increased emotional stability, increased imagination, and increased self-sufficiency."

But exercise has another intoxicating effect, which we mentioned in the chapter on exercise. It is thought that the exertion of exercise prompts the body to release endorphins, which are naturally-occurring opium-like substances. These can lead to an incredible euphoria which is known as "runner's high." As runner Ian Jackson related one endorphin-induced experience, "My senses were incredibly heightened, finely tuned in. I felt a natural unity with the dark trees and the drifting mist." So profound is this experience that Tom Jardin, psychologist and chemical-abuse counselor, recommends strenuous exercise as a safe way to turn off stress and get high.

There's another way to a natural high: deep relaxation. This may involve anything from a walk in the park to a period of Transcendental Meditation, but it all involves slowing the cycles of brain activity.

Your brain operates at four different "speeds": alpha, beta, theta and delta. In a waking state, the brain waves flow at 13 to 32 cycles per second, and this is known as the beta state. During moderate sleep, the brain operates at the theta state, or four to eight cycles per second. In deep sleep the brain slows to one-half to four cycles per second, and this is known as delta. However, at eight to 13 cycles per second the brain functions in a special way. It becomes more creative, more aware. This state is known as alpha. The goal of all deep relaxation activities is to slow the brain to this alpha state.

There are very many ways to attain this alpha state. Perhaps the most direct is biofeedback, in which a person hooks him- or herself up to a machine which monitors and reports the quality of brain waves. It is said that by becoming aware of one's brain energy in this fashion, it becomes possible to learn to lower oneself to the alpha state. This might work, but it sounds like a pretty high-tech way of getting high.

Meditation techniques are another path to alpha. These are usually detailed strategies for calming the body and becoming more conscious of one's surroundings. They include Transcendental Meditation, Relaxation Response, Autogenic Training, Progressive Relaxation and various forms of yoga and Zen. They may sound pretty weird, but most of them are fairly simple. Other people simply think of themselves in a calming, beautiful place—and there are a lot of other methods. You could probably develop your own, if you gave it some thought.

Meditation is thought to slow the metabolism and heart and respiration rates, lower blood acidity and support processes connected to the sympathetic nervous system. Best of all, it increases the likelihood and duration of alpha brain-wave cycles, and reduces muscle tension. It may be the best non-narcotic way to beat stress yet.

I suppose my own recommendation for getting high and beating stress is to make a definite effort to be creative in life. Take time to do the things that are important and rewarding to you. Explore your world. Sharpen your senses. Don't let yourself get caught in a deadening rut. After

all is said and done, you have one abiding
obligation to yourself. You owe it to yourself to
live.

13

MIRACLE MENU PLAN

The Miracle Menu Plan satisfies the body's hunger with minimal calories, keeps you from feeling hungry for hours, and helps you to feel great.

Very few menu plans can meet even one of these criteria, to say nothing of meeting all three. The Miracle Menu Plan frees you from kitchen drudgery and lets you spend more time doing what you enjoy. The menu plan cuts down on the time you need to prepare food for meals, as well as the time required to clean up afterwards—and time is money!

One of the secrets of the success of the Miracle Menu Plan is that it avoids appetite stimulants and addictive foods. White sugar, salt, refined white flour and fat all drive you to eat too much. In the Miracle Menu Plan, all such additives are avoided. When you first try the Plan, you may miss these harmful appetite stimulants, but in a short time you'll begin to discover the luscious, delicate flavors of whole, natural foods.

The foods recommended in the Miracle Menu Plan are designed to expand and pass through the stomach slowly. Modern super-refined foods have all the bulk taken out of them, so that you need to eat a lot to feel satisfied. The foods in the Miracle Menu Plan, though, stick with you, so you'll eat less often and feel more satisfied.

When you eat your food is almost as important as the amount that you eat. If you eat your largest meal just before watching TV or going to bed, your body can't do anything else than convert most of that food to fat and store it in undesirable places. If you eat your largest meal a few hours before the most active part of the day, your body will use the food as fuel to give you lots of energy, instead of converting it to fat. We've seen people get fat on 1000 calories a day because they would consume it as one meal just before going to bed, convert it to fat and they'd feel sluggish the next day.

You'll notice that, in the Miracle Menu Plan, the biggest meal of each day is breakfast. It's crucial to start the day with a nutritionally sound breakfast, since the way you feel in the morning affects how you'll feel all day. Also, you'll have a full day to metabolize all those calories. Lunches in the Plan are medium-sized, and suppers are the lightest. Snacking on the right foods is OK, too.

The Miracle Menu Plan requires that all foods be natural, because of their high nutrient content and complete flavor profile. Stay away from synthetic or "diet" foods, because they stimulate the appetite and do little to satisfy hunger.

One of the most important nutritional

components of the Miracle Menu Plan is bread. The breads I recommend are scientifically selected to be of such high nutritional value that they will provide the nutrients one normally gets from meat, potatoes, cooked vegetables and white bread. The Miracle Menu Plan will not work for you if you don't use the suggested breads, or very similar ones. Ordinary breads are much too low in nutritional value, and have little fiber, flavor or texture. The appetite stimulants and other chemical additives used in regular bread make it unsuitable for the plan. The breads I suggest are the sort of breads you can live on. Don't even attempt to live on white bread!

Despite my insistence on the right kind of bread, I don't want you to think that the Miracle Menu Plan is some sort of tyrannical program. Experiment with it, have fun with it. As long as you follow the general guidelines I discuss in this book, you can have a great deal of flexibility with the Plan.

Many so-called diet plans are harmful because they restrict food intake so severely that nutritional deficiencies may occur. If this happens, a person ends up feeling weak, depressed, dizzy, hungry and tired much of the time. I've never known this to happen to a person on the Miracle Menu Plan, but if it happens to you, consult your doctor. When followed conscientiously, the Plan will help people with heart trouble, hypoglycemia, diabetes, obesity, gall bladder trouble, arthritis or constipation. The plan will also help athletes, but they may want to increase the size of meals a bit. Let me stress again, however, that absolutely no junk foods should be eaten by a person on the Miracle Menu Plan.

The prepared foods listed in the Plan are made by Natural Ovens of Manitowoc, Wisconsin. When I mention Natural Ovens, I'm doing more than just selling my own product. Natural Ovens is a philosophy. It is one of the few companies I that tests its products on animals for safety and nutritional value. As I've already mentioned, this sort of animal testing is rare in the food industry, so Natural Ovens products are the only foods I can recommend wholeheartedly. If you don't have a Natural Ovens distributor in your area, I've included recipes for our products at the end of this section.

On this diet plan, you should be sure to drink plenty of water, both with and between meals. You should drink a large glass before each meal, and another between meals. It is best to consume the water at room temperature, but refrigerated water is acceptable. Any kind of water is good, but artesian water is best. Club soda or Perrier are acceptable, but they are no better for you and are rather expensive.

Food supplements may or may not be needed, depending on your individual requirements. If you're already taking a food supplement, you should stick with it. Then you might try experimenting to see if they are still needed. You may very well find that after a while on this high-nutrition plan you no longer need the same level of food supplements.

Some of you who have read *Fighting The Food Giants* will notice that this version of the Miracle Menu Plan is a bit different. I've modified the original plan to include more fiber and fewer calories.

Miracle Menu Plan
DAY ONE

Breakfast ½ Grapefruit, sectioned from top to bottom. Be sure to eat all the pulp. Two slices Sunny Millet Bread® with 1 tbls. natural peanut butter. Raspberry or red clover herbal tea (no caffeine)

Lunch   Two slices Sunny Millet Bread® with aged cheese melted on top. 1 cup fruit juice.

Supper   1 cup home made vegetable soup, your choice, with 4 tablespoons FIBRAN®. l cup cooked brown rice. Herb tea.

DAY TWO

Breakfast 4 tablespoons Pecan Granola® with milk and 2 tablespoons FIBRAN®. 1 slice Happiness Bread® or essene bread. 1 whole orange.

Lunch   Two slices Happiness Bread® or
               essene bread with cream cheese or
               butter.
               Tossed salad with 2 tablespoons
               any dressing.
               4. oz. broiled white fish.
Supper   One plate of steamed vegetables
               with 2 oz. melted cheese and 4
               tablespoons FIBRAN® over one
               slice of Sunny Millet Bread®.
               1 whole apple.

DAY THREE

Breakfast   Two ounces of cooked Happy Day
               Cereal with dried apple.
               Herb tea with 1 tablespoon honey.
Lunch   2 ounces veal liver (lightly cooked
               with onions).
               1 slice Sunny Millet Bread® with
               melted cheese.
               1 cup tomato juice.
Supper   One slice 100% Whole Grain Bread®
               or Brownberry's Health Nut® bread
               Small salad with 1 tablespoon your
               choice of dressing and 2 tablespoons
               FIBRAN®.
               Herb tea or fruit juice.
               Good Bite (sugar free) Cookie®.

DAY FOUR

Breakfast Sesame seeds sprinkled over fresh
pineapple
Herb tea Lunch
Small mixed vegetable salad
1 cup brown rice
4 oz. broiled ocean fish.
Pear.

Supper Cup of home made vegetable soup
with 4 tablespoons FIBRAN®.
½ cup brown rice.
Raspberry or red clover herbal tea
with 1 tablespoon honey.

DAY FIVE

Breakfast Diced pears with 2 tablespoons
sunflower seeds.
1 cup of grapefruit juice.

Lunch Large vegetable salad and 2
tablespoons choice of dressing, with
strips of aged cheese.
Herb tea.

Supper 1 cup lentil soup.
Steamed vegetables and tofu over
brown rice.
Mancha twig tea.

DAY SIX

Breakfast Heated whole wheat bun with 1 pat
           of butter.
           4 tablespoons Granola with milk
           and 2 tablespoons FIBRAN®, with
           ½ banana sliced in.
Lunch   Large salad with 2 tablespoons
           FIBRAN®, 3 tablespoons yogurt
           dressing.
           One slice Sunny Millet Bread® or
           essene bread with natural peanut
           butter.
           4. oz. veal liver
Supper   Small salad.
           Steamed vegetables with tofu.
           Brown rice with miso.
           Herb tea.

DAY SEVEN

Breakfast 4 ounces cooked Happy Day Cereal®
           with prunes.
           1 cup milk.
           1 cup Herb Tea.
Lunch   Fresh fruit salad.
           1 slice Sunny Millet Bread®.
           or Brownberry's Health Nut® bread
           1 cup hot cider or fruit juice.
Supper   Vegetarian salad with 2 tablespoons
           your choice of dressing.
           1 Whole wheat bun.
           1 glass grapefruit juice.

If you suffer from distressing hunger between meals, you may snack on high-fiber mixtures of seeds and nuts, such as Sunshine Snack Mix® or Punch Snack Mix®. Drink plenty of water (we recommend Mountain Valley Water).

It's important that you try to minimize snacking after 8 p.m., as this will hinder your appetite for a good breakfast the next morning.

®Registered Trademark of Natural Ovens, 1926 South 9th Street, Manitowoc, Wisconsin 54220.

Sunny Millet Bread

Oil	2 tbls.	Whole wheat flour	1 cup
Honey	2 tbls.	Gluten flour	2 cups
Water	2½ cups	Rolled oats	2 cups
Yeast (moist)	1 oz.	Salt	2 tsp.
Sunflower seeds	¼ cup	Barley malt	1 tsp.
Cracked wheat	½ cup	Sesame seeds	3 tsp.
		Millet	¼ cup

Mix all ingredients at once. Knead for 10 minutes. Should be slightly sticky. Let rise, cover with a board, 1 hr. Punch down, wait 15 min., form into 2 loaves. Work out all possible air. Allow to double (not higher than ½" below the top of a regular loaf pan). Bake at 350° approximately 30 min. in the oven. Grease pan lightly before baking. Loaf should be 3½" high by 8" long and weigh about 1½ lbs. NOTE: It is very important to use high gluten flour so that the flour has enough strength to rise with heavy seeds in it.

Scotch Oaties Cookies

Butter (melted)	1 lb.	Raw sugar	2 lbs.
Eggs	6	Whole wheat flour	3 cups
Oil	⅔ cup	Gluten flour	3 cups
Vanilla	1 tbls.	Rolled oats	8 cups
Honey	1 lb.	Baking soda	¼ tsp.
Water	2 cups	Cinnamon	¾ tsp.
(more or less)		Nutmeg	¼ tsp.
Lemon extract	1 tbls.	Buttermilk pwdr.	1 cup

Mix together with electric mixer on medium speed butter, raw sugar, eggs, oil, vanilla and honey. Mix dry ingredients together and then add liquids.

Bake at 320° about 12 minutes on cookie sheet (lightly greased). Makes plenty.

Happiness Bread

Honey	¼ cup	Malt	1 tsp.
Oil	3 tbls.	Potato flour	1 tbls.
Yeast (cake)	2 oz.	Pecan pieces	2 tbls.
Water	3¼ cups	Cinnamon	1 tsp.
Whole wheat flour	2½ cups	Raisins	1 cup
Gluten flour	2½ cups	Rolled oats	1 cup
		Salt	½ tsp.

Mix all ingredients except pecan pieces, cinnamon, and raisins. Mix for 12 minutes.

Then evenly distribute nuts, raisins, and cinnamon. Should be slightly sticky. Let rise an hour. Punch down and let rest for 15 minutes. Knead. Divide into two loaves. Second time let double in size in loaf pan. 350°. Bake 30-40 min. Lightly grease loaf pan. Loaf should weigh 1½ lb. Size should be approximately 4" high and 8" long after baking. Should sound hollow when thumped on the bottom.

Fibran

Vanilla	1 tbls.	Wheat germ	1 lb.
Lecithin	3 oz.	Barley malt	3 oz.
Bran	3 lb.	Cinnamon	1 tbls.

Mix in mixer 5 minutes. (Do not use blender).

Sunshine Snack Mix

Mix all ingredients together in large bowl.

Raw sunflower seeds	11 oz.
Salted sunflower seeds	8 oz.
Salted cashews	4 oz.
Raisins	5 oz.
Salted almonds	4 oz.

Gourmet Snack Mix

Mix together in a large bowl.

Raw deluxe nuts	10 oz.
Cocktail peanuts	10 oz.
Raisins	4 oz.
Apricots	6 oz.

Pecan Granola

Oil	6 oz.
Honey	6 oz.
Vanilla	1 tbls.

Rolled oats	2 lbs.	Bran	4 oz.
Coconut	3 oz.	Sesame seeds	1 oz.
Wheat germ	3 oz.	Cinnamon	2 tsp.
Salt	dash	Pecans	4 oz.
Sunflower seeds	3 oz.		

Mix together in large bowl. Mix by hand, rolled oats, coconut, wheat germ, sunflower seeds, bran, sesame seeds and then add the rest of ingredients.

Spread on cookie sheet, thin and evenly. Bake at 325°. Bake 10 min. (Watch closely until toasted lightly).

Happy Days Cereal

Rolled barley	8 oz.
Steel cut oats	8 oz.
Sesame seeds	1 oz.
Sunflower seeds	2 oz.

Whole Wheat Buns

Warm water	3 cups	Oat flour	⅔ cups
Granulated yeast	2 tbsp.	Potato flour	1 tbsp.
Malt	5 tbsp.	Salt	2 tsp.
Gluten flour	3¾ cups	Soy Oil	5 tbsp.
Whole wheat flour	3¾ cups		

2 dozen buns

Have all ingredients room temperature!

Dissolve the yeast and malt in warm water. Add salt, soy oil, potato flour, oat flour and gluten flour. Mix well. Add whole wheat flour, but one cup. Turn the dough on to floured board. Add rest of whole wheat flour and knead for 10 minutes. Place in oiled bowl. Cover the dough with a damp cloth and allow to rise until doubled about 60 minutes. Punch down and let raise for 1 more hour. Punch down. Shape into 24 buns. Cover with damp cloth and let rise until double, about 40 minutes. Bake in preheated oven, 350 degrees for 20-25 minutes. Cool on rack.

100% Whole Wheat Bread

Water	3½ cups	Oat flour	1 cup
Granulated Yeast	2 tbsp.	Salt	2 tsp.
Malt	¼ cup	Soy oil	¼ cup
Whole wheat flour	7 cups	Egg	1
Wheat Germ	⅔ cup		

2 Loaves

Have all ingredients room temperature!

Dissolve the yeast and malt in warm water. Add salt, soy oil, egg, oat flour and half the whole wheat flour. Knead on a lightly floured board until the dough is pliable and soft (about 10 to 15 minutes). Shape into ball and place in an oiled bowl. Turn to coat the dough. Cover the bowl with a damp cloth and allow to rise until doubled about 60 minutes. Punch down dough and let raise for 1 more hour. After second raising shape into 2 loaves. Place in oiled loaf pans. Cover with damp cloth and let rise until double, 50-60 minutes. Bake in preheated oven, 350 degrees for 50-60 minutes. Cool on rack.

NUTRITIONAL GUIDELINES FOR THE COUNSELOR

Strategies for using metabolic correction to treat emotional and behavorial disorders

Barbara J. Reed's work with metabolic correction as Chief Probation Officer of the Municipal Court of Cuyahoga Falls, Ohio, has won her national attention. Now Reed provides educators, probation and parole officers, psychologists, social workers and all those in the counseling professions with a proven system for evaluating and correcting the physical problems which underlie many behavorial and emotions disorders.

In *Nutritional Guidelines for the Counselor,* Reed presents a clear, concise discussion of the links between diet and behavior, and describes how the nutritional approach has worked for others. She offers practical, detailed strategies for determining if a behavior problem has a metabolic root, and if so, what the counselor can do about it.

Included are tested screening questionnaires which the professional can use to discover if a dietary evaluation is indicated, and a thorough biography and contact list.

Just $10.00 (plus $2.00 postage and handling) from:

NATURAL PRESS
P.O. Box 2107
Manitowoc, WI 54220

FIGHTING
THE
FOOD
GIANTS

FOOD, TEENS & BEHAVIOR

Can the things kids eat really affect the way they behave? The evidence says YES. Now, Barbara Reed, PhD, former probation officer and nationally recognized educator in the field of diet and behavior, shows how the typical teenage junk food diet can lead to learning disabilities, delinquency, and even criminal behavior.

A decade of distinguished research work in the criminal justice system has convinced Reed that the quality of brain nutrition has a profound impact on the functioning of the mind. She has developed THE MOST EFFECTIVE PROGRAM IN THE NATION TO KEEP PROBATIONERS FROM GETTING BACK INTO TROUBLE.

In FOOD, TEENS & BEHAVIOR, Reed examines the biochemical roots of delinquency and crime in easy-to-understand language. She also explains fully how to provide adolescents with the best possible brain nutrition — and how to keep them from becoming part of the millions of teenagers arrested in this country every year.

FOOD, TEENS & BEHAVIOR is a book for the parents of teens in trouble — and for those who want to help their children avoid trouble. It is also a valuable guide for anyone who works with young people, such as psychologists, probation officers and guidance counselors.

Just $7.00 (plus $2.00 postage and handling) from:

NATURAL PRESS
P.O. Box 2107
Manitowoc, WI 54220

YES! I WANT TO ORDER THESE EXCITING NATURAL PRESS PAPERBACKS TODAY!

Please send me:

_____ copies of *Fighting The Food Giants* ($5.00 plus $2.00 postage and handling each).

_____ copies of *Why Calories Don't Count* ($7.00 plus $2.00 postage and handling each).

_____ copies of *The Low Cost, No-Fuss, All-Natural Food Guide For Students* (And Other Desperate People) ($4.95 plus $1.00 postage and handling each).

_____ copies of *Food, Teens & Behavior* ($7.00 plus $2.00 postage and handling each).

_____ copies of *Nutritional Guidelines for the Counselor* ($10.00 plus $2.00 postage and handling each).

NATURAL PRESS
P.O. Box 2107, Manitowoc, WI 54220

I enclose _____ for the books ordered above.

Name _____

Address _____

City _____ State _____ Zip _____

ALLOW THREE WEEKS FOR DELIVERY